Age to Perfection

Stay Smart!
Luts all Age to
Perfection!

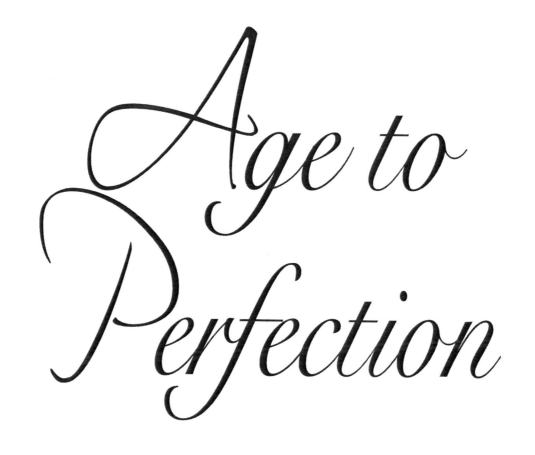

Age to Perfection

How to Thrive to 100, Happy, Healthy, and Wise

BY

J. MARK ANDERSON, MD, DABFM

WALTER GAMAN, MD, DABFM, FAAFP, FCFP

JUDITH K. GAMAN, BSHS, CCRC, CMA

Age to Perfection: How to Thrive to 100, Happy, Healthy, and Wise

Copyright © 2013 by J. Mark Anderson, Walter Gaman, and Judith K. Gaman.

George House Publishing

Library of Congress Control Number: 2013950064

ISBN: 978-0-9840731-2-2

Printed in the United States of America

CONTENTS

DEDICATIONS

I would like to dedicate this book to all people who want to live vibrantly until their last breath. Also, our staff at Executive Medicine has been so supportive of this whole process.

My partner Mark Anderson is the gentlest soul that I know—this book would be impossible without him.

I could not have done this without my wife Judy, who is the love and light of my life.

Je Ne Regrette Rien.

—WALTER GAMAN

This book is dedicated to all those who have gone before us and blazed our path to a century of living.

—MARK ANDERSON

During this process, I had the pleasure of interviewing the most amazing people. One in particular touched my heart and changed my life. I dedicate this book to Lucille Fleming, one of my favorite people of all time. At 100 years she is still full of life and an inspiration to not only me, but everyone who is blessed to know her.

—JUDY GAMAN

ACKNOWLEDGMENTS

It takes a team of dedicated people with a variety of talents to bring forth a final manuscript that educates and inspires the reader. We have been fortunate to work with some of the most committed, professional individuals in the industry. Couple that with interviewing some of the most fascinating people on this planet, and it makes for a great experience.

Our sincerest thanks to:

Emily Allen (Writing Assistant)—Your countless hours of editing and revising were done without complaint and always with a quirky smile. You are so talented and dedicated to the art of writing. Judy promises to make you Brazilian cheese balls whenever you want them during the course of the next 100 years.

Andrew Gaman (Illustrator)—We're not sure you knew just how many illustrations you were going to be signing up for. The first ones were so good that we just couldn't stop sending you more ideas. We are in awe of your many talents and infinite wisdom.

Brion Sausser (Book Design)—It has been pleasure to work with you again. We know we can always count on you to deliver a fantastic final product. You really are the BEST in this business.

Audra Gorgiev (Editor)—Thank you for working miracles, especially in a time crunch. You're amazing!

Sandy Peddicord (Publicist)—Not sure how many hats you could possibly wear. Not only are you a great publicist, but you have unsurpassed talents as a therapist. When things get tough…call Sandy! You are amazing, and we are very blessed to have you so invested in the success of this book.

Emme (Foreword)—You have been such a positive influence to so many people around the world; we are blessed and privileged to spend time with you. Thank you for your kind words and your vote of confidence.

The Staff of Executive Medicine of Texas—When we were wrapped up in this book, you kept the fires burning bright back at the office. You are a dedicated group of intelligent individuals who make it easy for us to do what we do best. May we always celebrate our successes together. We love all of you and are thrilled to have you on our team.

FOREWORD

I am absolutely delighted to write the foreword for *AGE TO PERFECTION: How to Thrive to 100, Happy Healthy and Wise.* The authors of this book truly know how to take the patients they treat to a higher level of wellness. Everyone needs hope, and I hope that the chapters of this book give you great insight into your own health and add years to your life.

Knowing that each person's journey is different, I love that this book addresses the need for personal responsibility from each and every one of us. As we all become more personally responsible for our health, we can enjoy all that life has to offer, without being weighed down by the burdens of diabetes, heart disease, and the like.

My introduction to Drs. Walter Gaman and Mark Anderson's thriving Executive Medicine of Texas practice couldn't have come at a better time for me. Just hours beforehand, I had found myself having a familiar—and frustrating—conversation with a producer and later on air with the anchor at a major network about me actually being very healthy despite my body mass index stating I was obese. As a model and spokesperson in the fashion industry for over 20 years, I've had to dispel the myth at least a few hundred times that thinness equates with fitness and health—a fallacy that continues to affect millions of people, especially women, forcing them to strive for an ideal of health that's clearly not their own, nor something they should ever attempt to attain. This in itself is very unhealthy! I felt then, as I do now, that society's unsound standards of health alienate millions of people *from* being healthy, leading to confusion, unhealthy practices, and premature death. So, when I visited Executive Medicine of Texas to undergo their Executive Physical, I quickly realized their unique mission. I saw that their practice honored the individual's health—not through a purely medical approach, but a preventative holistic one that included nutrients and micronutrients, consistent fitness, personal accountability, and balance. I knew I had finally found a kindred spirit, a place where I could arrive at real answers to my own health questions and possibly an avenue through which to credibly confront the currently held societal ideal. The results were both extremely validating and incredibly valuable. Everybody should have the opportunity to look at their body from the inside out! While I was ahead of the bell curve on health, I could still use some fine-tuning (couldn't we all?).

To quote Dr. Gaman: "If looking into a mirror could tell you everything you need to know about your health, a dressing room could do a physician's job. While body type and size play a role in health, I have seen many very thin people who are unhealthy on the inside, as well as larger outer appearances that have great internal health. Sometimes, fine tuning is all a body needs to add years to one's life."

This insight personally resonated with me, and provided a different perspective and level of justification about my body/health that had challenged me throughout my career. I felt empowered. It was then I knew I was going to speak up about what I learned, but this time with a doctor's stamp of approval.

I wanted to take action (and responsibility) for the additional 25 pounds I had allowed to creep up over the last 20 years (basically, a pound a year) since my being a size 12 at the beginning of my modeling career. I wanted to do it in a healthy way, but didn't want to catch heat from the size acceptance movement for "caving in" to the current unrealistic standards of beauty, which I felt my 25 extra pounds had nothing to do with. I was ready to put myself, Dr. G., and medicine to the test. My goal? To open minds of what another ideal of fitness and healthy can look like. Thankfully, I now have an internal road map outlining strengths and the areas that need attention. Being a single mom, I felt I had an obligation to my daughter and myself to address whatever I may need to know immediately, rather than live with the worry of the unknown. None of us should deny ourselves the best health and longest life possible!

Needless to say, I feel like I have a new lease on life. Now it's up to me to maintain it. I hope my life-changing experience encourages you to be open and take the first steps toward a happy, healthy and wise life for yourself.

Anyone interested in prolonging their life and improving their wellness stands to benefit from the proactive message of personal responsibility advocated by Drs. Gaman and Anderson. This is why I'm thrilled about *Age to Perfection*.

INTRODUCTION

As physicians, we have the privilege of delivering newborns, watching and feeling the first breath of life rush into the lungs, and hearing that first cry. Sometimes they need a little encouragement; a swift tap on the rear usually suffices. Fast forward several years, to the last breathe to leave the dying body, often quietly and without much fanfare. The span between the first inspiration and the last exhalation is what defines our quality of life. Time, events, accomplishments, and relationships define our very existence.

Quality of life begins with good health. In medicine, we are taught to diagnose and treat diseases. Some of us expand and build on that knowledge by seeking to transcend beyond reactionary healthcare, and become proactive by keeping the diseases from ever reaching the body.

Transcending tradition is not unique. Great thinkers have always shared the understanding that everything is connected, and seek insight by expanding their frame of reference. Da Vinci, Michelangelo, Rafael, and Machiavelli all looked outside of the norms of their field to change the very landscape of what they did. Through this process, a renaissance was born. From that point forward, all artists have seen their palettes differently.

Medicine is entering its own renaissance, as cellular and genetic information is reframing our perception on not only how to treat disease, but how to prevent it. Genetic evaluation can now predict prevalence for disease. Just as the revivals of classical Greek and Roman thought propelled the cultural movement of the Renaissance, these medical advances propel modern science forward. We now have access to medical advancements that our grandparents would never have thought possible; likewise, the healthcare opportunities of our children and grandchildren will far exceed our wildest expectations.

In the following chapters, we bring you a concise and readable synopsis of how you can take full advantage of modern, forward-thinking science. We are able to share this advice with our patients on a daily basis, as we help promote longevity and vitality. Good health often requires revision and repetition; identifying weaknesses, and instating good habits. Some of what we discuss is old news (sometimes centuries old), while some has yet to hit medical textbooks. We seek to educate, motivate, and perhaps entertain you, as you begin your journey to better health and a longer life.

In good health,

—J. Mark Anderson, MD

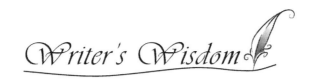

THE TENTH-FLOOR BALCONY

During the course of writing this book, I retreated to the Adolphus Hotel in Dallas, Texas, so that I could catch up on writing, as the deadline was fast approaching. It's amazing what happens to the brain when it has downtime to regenerate with original ideas and new inspiration. In today's society, we are often so suffocated with information that sometimes it's hard to even breathe. Our cell phones, and televisions, along with work and home schedules all overwhelm our senses, leaving little room for self-revelation.

After a long period of contemplation about the manuscript and the realization that I had left out a critical piece of context, I retreated to the balcony of my tenth-story hotel room for some fresh air. Not only did I get fresh air, I got a new perspective on life. Leaning over the balcony, I looked to both my left and right and came to a unique conclusion about our time on earth.

The Adolphus sits on Commerce Street in downtown Dallas, a busy area with lots of hustle and bustle. Cars, pedestrians, and bicyclists fill the street. Looking from my perch in the sky, I could see a highway on each side about a mile out, with me almost directly in the middle. Suddenly, I realized that Commerce Street reminds me of life. Sometimes we stop and sometimes we go, just like the cars waiting in the intersections.

The business of life is our Commerce Street, filling the space between the highways that lead us to our biggest successes or greatest challenges. As we go about our daily business, we have to decide to take the on-ramp or simply go under the overpass, continuing with the stop-and-go humdrum that we have grown accustomed to. Any one of the highways we are given could lead us to a whole new place in life. Sometimes that place is filled with happiness and great opportunities, and sometimes it's filled with pain or disappointment, but we have to take highways that represent a little bit of both before we can reach our final destination.

Regardless of which stretch of the road we are on, sometimes a pit stop is in order. I encourage everyone to find their own "tenth-floor balcony" and reflect on life. Take a moment to regenerate and let your heart seek personal revelation. If you do, the highways won't sneak up quite as fast, and even if they do, you'll be prepared for the on-ramp.

—Judy Gaman

CHAPTER ONE

PERSONAL RESPONSIBILITY

It's up to you to save yourself

> "The way you think, the way you behave, the way you eat, can influence your life by 30 to 50 years." —Deepak Chopra

At no other time in the history of the United States has there been so much debate over healthcare. Our country is divided between the previously accepted third-party payer system and extensive governmental takeover of the healthcare system. In 2010, health expenditures in the United States reached almost $2.6 trillion, which is over 10 times the $256 billion spent three decades prior. Of the $2.6 trillion, 51% of that was spent on hospital and physician office visits. It's easy to blame the rising cost of healthcare on increases in premiums, but the real expense lies in the vast time and energy being devoted to the treatment of so many preventable diseases.

The nation may continue to squabble over who is ultimately responsible for rising healthcare costs, but at the end of the day, the answer remains the same: you and I are responsible. The only real way to lower costs for disease management is to avoid getting the diseases in the first place. While we recognize that some diseases may be unavoidable, at least at this point in time, most illnesses and deaths occur as a result of poor personal choices.

Do you know the culprit behind much of the disease, disability, and death that plague this country? When we ask our patients this question, we get all sorts of answers—and over 90% of the time, their answers are wrong. If you have ever walked through a cloud of smoke while an employee of your favorite store sits outside puffing away on a cigarette, then you, too, have been exposed to the number one killer in the United States: tobacco. Annually, over 443,000 people die prematurely from exposure to cigarette smoke, either directly or through the negligence of a smoking parent, child, spouse, or acquaintance. When you put this tragedy into dollars and cents, it amounts to $96 billion a year in medical costs, plus an additional $97 billion in lost wages and productivity. To comprehend the magnitude of this loss, imagine a city roughly the size of Sacramento, California, being wiped out year after year. As a nation, we build memorials honoring lives lost due to tragedy, which in number is only a fraction of the amount of lives lost to tobacco. The true tragedy of our time is largely ignored.

> *INSTANT*INSIGHT Genetics play a small role in heart attacks. Healthy lifestyle choices, such as the decision to eat well, can decrease the likelihood of heart attack or stroke by as much as 80%. Fighting cardiovascular disease doesn't have to mean overcoming genetics. It can be as simple as the few choices we make every day. Imagine a world where more people took this advice to heart.

Often the things that cause us the most grief in life are self-induced. Time and time again, patients develop diabetes, heart disease, or cancer and wonder how they ever got to that point. Most diseases just don't happen overnight, but progress gradually, going unnoticed until it is too late. Fortunately, it doesn't have to be this way. Taking time to understand your health risks and then dedicating your life to healthy choices going forward will make a difference. That difference may just save your life.

Preventative and proactive medicine is changing the landscape of healthcare by allowing patients to take charge of their own health concerns. Comparing your health metrics yearly—such as body mass index (BMI), cholesterol, and blood pressure—may change the course of your destiny and rewrite your life's ending. If your goal is to live to 100 happy, healthy, and wise—then this book can help you do that. Notice that we say *help*. This book cannot do it for you, because it is you that must take action. You must take personal responsibility—it really is up to you to save yourself!

It's Not Too Late

Once, a 62-year-old male patient, Jim, came in asking if it was "too late" for him. He had fallen deeply in love for the second time in his life and suddenly felt he had something to live for again. Since the death of his late wife, he had gained almost 100 pounds, started drinking each night, and had given up on exercise altogether. Jim was nothing short of a train wreck. Not only did he look tired and worn, he had poor circulation and had developed type 2 diabetes. He made the choice to take charge of his health and get his life back on track. Within six months, Jim lost 50 pounds, his blood sugars were close to normal levels, and he looked like a new man—one fit for a bride.

Whether you are 20, 50, or even 80 years old, it's never too late to take charge—just like Jim did—and make positive changes. The sooner you do, the better your long-term outcome will be. Don't waste energy focusing on past mistakes. Maybe you have a history of drug use, alcohol abuse, or overeating. Your past shouldn't determine your attitude about your future. Healthy choices made today will help repair the damage of yesterday.

> "Character—the willingness to accept responsibility for one's own life—is the source from which self-respect springs." —Joan Didion, *On Self-Respect*

Mental and Emotional Shape

Taking responsibility for your health is more than just about reaching your ideal weight or avoiding toxic habits. It's about paying attention to all aspects of your being. Emotional, physical, and spiritual health each require regular maintenance. A healthy body is a sign of a person who is well maintained in all areas.

If you find yourself on an emotional roller coaster, determine the source of your turmoil and find your way back to sanity. This may require some help from your healthcare provider, so don't be afraid to discuss what's going on inside your head. A runaway mind can be the root cause of many health issues. Remember, if everyone is getting on your nerves, the problem probably isn't with everyone else. In the words of Michael Jackson: "Start with the man in the mirror." Choosing to address your emotional problems and taking time to find the root causes of them will not only save your sanity, it may also save your job, marriage, and other relationships.

If symptoms persist, seek help. Some forms of depression or anger are signs of a separate health concern. If you are experiencing changes in your mental or emotional status, be sure to have a complete physical exam. While medications such as antidepressants may be necessary, they shouldn't be a Band-Aid that covers up the underlying issue. Psychological problems should never be analyzed in isolation from your overall health. A complete physical examination and laboratory assessment should be used to eliminate any other medical reasons for depression or anxiety. For example, medical issues like sleep apnea and certain vitamin deficiencies can cause psychological changes. With 1 in 10 adults in the United States suffering from depression, the antidepressant market has grown exponentially. Our goal is to determine the root cause of the symptoms and work toward a healthy body, free of unnecessary medication. When medications are indicated, they should be taken for an appropriate amount of time.

Physical Shape

As you age, maintaining good physical condition will help prevent injury and illness. Fitness is defined differently for each of us. Not everyone can, or should, run a marathon. However, each person has the responsibility to stay physically fit and as healthy as possible, within the context of their body type.

Gaining weight and losing muscle mass are no big mystery. If you eat too much, you gain weight. If you don't get moving and exercise your body, you will not only gain weight, you will lose muscle mass.

"I don't know why I can't lose this weight" is a complaint heard by doctors all over the country day in and day out. With the exception of certain uncommon medical conditions, the recipe for good health is simple: eat nutritiously, exercise regularly, and get enough sleep. This simple solution is available to everyone, regardless of race, age, sex, or socioeconomic status. However, it requires a great amount of self-discipline from the individual. Those who take good care of their body increase the chance for living a longer life.

OUT OF THE MOUTHS OF BABES

Most of us have an innate sense of what it takes to get and stay healthy. At the end of this book, we reveal advice from centenarians on what they feel is necessary for living a long and healthy life. Here, we consulted with those at the other end of the age spectrum, and they did not disappoint! The following is a fun look at what the youngest generation had to say when asked "What does it take to get to your 100th birthday?"

AVYONNE JONES, AGE 9

Eat healthy, exercise, replenish your bones, and nap a lot.

LINDSEY TRUE, AGE 8

You take a special pill with strawberry ice cream. Don't get fat and get a face-lift like my grandma Honey.

REAGAN OHEARN, AGE 11

Drink a glass of wine every day.

TIM OHEARN, AGE 9

Grow your own crops.

TOM OHEARN, AGE 8

Be happy.

BADEN CHINN, AGE 10

Eat healthy.

ELLA MOORE, AGE 4

I can't even count to 100 because then I wouldn't be able to sleep. Those old people do not get in trouble. They do not get in the road. They don't break a rule 'cause they're just nice.

EMMELINE MOORE, AGE 9

Well, we can all learn to be 100. It's just that we each have different problems to get there because we are all different. I think you need to be strong, wise, and kind. It's not your fault if you die young.

HEATHER FARMER, AGE 11

Well, first off…I will try anything to keep me alive. I will try vegetables, fruit, vitamins…good and healthy vitamins for my heart and brain, like my grandma and grandpa take. And I'll take advice from really good friends. I will eat prunes everyday because I won't have any teeth. I'm going to try to stay as healthy as possible, and be the best I can be. I'll be a good person and won't get in trouble. And just treat God the way you're supposed to be treated and hopefully your wish will be true.

TIFFANY FARMER, AGE 11

Love your mom, and, um, just keep yourself in the food pyramid. Also, take your vitamins each day, like you're supposed to, and eat healthy things, like I just said. And just try your best to get some exercise each day, like a five minute walk or something, and make sure you do healthy things for your body. Eat an apple a day, 'cause you know what they say, 'An apple a day keeps the doctor away.' Also, being old means life is going to be fun for you, because you have lots of experience.

COURTNEY FARMER, AGE 6

Eat a lot of healthy food, and seeing the doctor of course, because you're old. Old ladies don't get any help, but sometimes they do, and I love my Mommy, and that's it.

NICK GUNIAVA, AGE 2

(How old do you want to be someday?) He extends both hands to the sky and says, *This tall!* (How will you get that old?) *By eating.*

For the most part, these responses are spot on: eat right, get adequate sleep, stay safe, and control your weight. Something happens between childhood and early adulthood that that makes us lose sight of basic health principles. Maybe it's advertising or peer pressure, or maybe we just get too busy to care. However, if we can hold on to our natural proclivity toward good health and keep our focus on making positive choices, the chance of being around to see our great-great-grandchildren improves dramatically.

"I'm not much but I'm all I have." —Philip K. Dick, *Martian Time-Slip*

Responsibility = Freedom

Imagine living far into the second half of your life without the burden of failing health, large medical bills, or limited mobility. Many people are living fulfilling lives to their 100th birthday and beyond. Living a long and healthy life is possible, and it's not really as hard as some people may think. Good health is the key to freedom, because nothing makes us freer than having personal independence.

> ***INSTANT*INSIGHT** Did you know the bad habits you develop early in life could affect generations to come? A new field of study called epigenomics is unlocking the mysteries behind inherited mutations. Protect your own DNA and that of future generations by making good, healthy lifestyle choices *before* you have children.

Good health brings freedom that isn't just a benefit for the individual, but a benefit to the family. The relationships between adult children and their parents look very different depending on the amount of care and support that the parents require. If the parents have maintained a healthy lifestyle and have had the good fortune to not to fall victim to health concerns beyond their control, the last decades of their life will be filled with great bonding and mentoring opportunities. On the contrary, an unhealthy elderly parent can drain the adult child emotionally, physically, and mentally. In the event that a parent's failing health is due to bad personal choices such as smoking, drinking, poor diet, or a sedentary lifestyle, then the adult child may also feel resentment. The stress brought on by this resentment can cause health problems for both the caregiver and the parent being cared for.

As we have said many times over in this book, good health is the result of good choices. Each day that your feet hit the floor, you should rise with a smile on your face and a grateful attitude for the good fortune of living another day. Let your daily routine be a monument to your vitality and gratitude.

> ***INSTANT*INSIGHT** Keep it POSITIVE! Being happy with your age will help you age better. After 23 years of research, scientists at Yale University found that having a positive attitude toward the aging process increases longevity by 7.5 years.

Ten Ways You Can Be Responsible

1. Eat a healthy, balanced diet full of fresh fruits and vegetables.
2. Avoid fried food and processed carbohydrates.
3. Avoid toxins like tobacco and alcohol.
4. Find some time each day to exercise.
5. Avoid watching more than one hour of television per day.
6. Take charge of your thought life and avoid negativity.
7. Keep your BMI at a reasonable number.
8. Drink plenty of water.
9. Pay attention to warning signs that your body gives you (medical intuition).
10. Get a yearly physical exam.

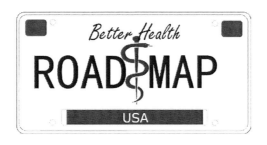

Body Mass Index Table

	Normal						Overweight					Obese										Extreme Obesity														
BMI	19	20	21	22	23	24	25	26	27	28	29	30	31	32	33	34	35	36	37	38	39	40	41	42	43	44	45	46	47	48	49	50	51	52	53	54
Height (inches)																	Body Weight (pounds)																			
58	91	96	100	105	110	115	119	124	129	134	138	143	148	153	158	162	167	172	177	181	186	191	196	201	205	210	215	220	224	229	234	239	244	248	253	258
59	94	99	104	109	114	119	124	128	133	138	143	148	153	158	163	168	173	178	183	188	193	198	203	208	212	217	222	227	232	237	242	247	252	257	262	267
60	97	102	107	112	118	123	128	133	138	143	148	153	158	163	168	174	179	184	189	194	199	204	209	215	220	225	230	235	240	245	250	255	261	266	271	276
61	100	106	111	116	122	127	132	137	143	148	153	158	164	169	174	180	185	190	195	201	206	211	217	222	227	232	238	243	248	254	259	264	269	275	280	285
62	104	109	115	120	126	131	136	142	147	153	158	164	169	175	180	186	191	196	202	207	213	218	224	229	235	240	246	251	256	262	267	273	278	284	289	295
63	107	113	118	124	130	135	141	146	152	158	163	169	175	180	186	191	197	203	208	214	220	225	231	237	242	248	254	259	265	270	278	282	287	293	299	304
64	110	116	122	128	134	140	145	151	157	163	169	174	180	186	192	197	204	209	215	221	227	232	238	244	250	256	262	267	273	279	285	291	296	302	308	314
65	114	120	126	132	138	144	150	156	162	168	174	180	186	192	198	204	210	216	222	228	234	240	246	252	258	264	270	276	282	288	294	300	306	312	318	324
66	118	124	130	136	142	148	155	161	167	173	179	186	192	198	204	210	216	223	229	235	241	247	253	260	266	272	278	284	291	297	303	309	315	322	328	334
67	121	127	134	140	146	153	159	166	172	178	185	191	198	204	211	217	223	230	236	242	249	255	261	268	274	280	287	293	299	306	312	319	325	331	338	344
68	125	131	138	144	151	158	164	171	177	184	190	197	203	210	216	223	230	236	243	249	256	262	269	276	282	289	295	302	308	315	322	328	335	341	348	354
69	128	135	142	149	155	162	169	176	182	189	196	203	209	216	223	230	236	243	250	257	263	270	277	284	291	297	304	311	318	324	331	338	345	351	358	365
70	132	139	146	153	160	167	174	181	188	195	202	209	216	222	229	236	243	250	257	264	271	278	285	292	299	306	313	320	327	334	341	348	355	362	369	376
71	136	143	150	157	165	172	179	186	193	200	208	215	222	229	236	243	250	257	265	272	279	286	293	301	308	315	322	329	338	343	351	358	365	372	379	386
72	140	147	154	162	169	177	184	191	199	206	213	221	228	235	242	250	258	265	272	279	287	294	302	309	316	324	331	338	346	353	361	368	375	383	390	397
73	144	151	159	166	174	182	189	197	204	212	219	227	235	242	250	257	265	272	280	288	295	302	310	318	325	333	340	348	355	363	371	378	386	393	401	408
74	148	155	163	171	179	186	194	202	210	218	225	233	241	249	256	264	272	280	287	295	303	311	319	326	334	342	350	358	365	373	381	389	396	404	412	420
75	152	160	168	176	184	192	200	208	216	224	232	240	248	256	264	272	279	287	295	303	311	319	327	335	343	351	359	367	375	383	391	399	407	415	423	431
76	156	164	172	180	189	197	205	213	221	230	238	246	254	263	271	279	287	295	304	312	320	328	336	344	353	361	369	377	385	394	402	410	418	426	435	443

GLADYS REEVES, 90.5 YEARS YOUNG, TORRANCE, CALIFORNIA

During the 37 years of her life as a counselor in the Long Beach school system, she learned the importance of being positive, even when it's hard to do. She has always avoided smoking, secondhand smoke, and alcohol. She still lives in the house they built back in 1952. "Have a large circle of friends to laugh and share life's challenges with. I loves going to concerts and taking in all that life has to offer."

CHAPTER TWO

THE AGING SYNDROME

Time and our bodies

"Count your age by friends, not years. Count your
life by smiles, not tears." —John Lennon

It takes about 20 years from birth for the body to reach its highest potential for overall health. By that time, hormones have leveled out and the brain is functioning at full capacity. The prime years between 20 and 30 are the best years to be focusing on good habits and creating a positive imprint on the body for years to come. This is also the time that a body has the most potential for physical strength. Once the body reaches about 40 years of age, it starts changing, and if not properly prepared, it can become vulnerable to disease and begin to age very quickly.

Each individual will age chronologically the same way—another year, another candle on the cake. On the flip side, the biological progression of aging is vastly different from person to person. How the body's health declines is a combination of genetic and environmental factors, as well as the lifestyle choices that are made, such as nutrition and exercise. This is why you see "old" 60-year-olds and "young" 90-year-olds.

While it is not our goal to play God, or achieve immortality, it is very much our goal to help people understand how the aging process works. We want them to embrace longevity with more candles on the cake and a sparkle in their eyes. Everyone will age with time, but "old" is starting to look very different than the "old" of a few generations ago. The choices made throughout life can greatly change a person's health and happiness forecast.

For the first two decades of life, the body is in an anabolic state, constantly constructive, each day becoming bigger and better. Imagine the construction of a large object with Lego, each additional piece adding to a greater and more complex whole. This is what happens during the years from birth through college age. For the next two decades, as adulthood sets in, the carefully constructed masterpiece is in a plateau with no real additions or changes. However, at about 40 years from the beginning of construction, small pieces start to fall off, some pieces may crack with age, and the structure loses its newness and some of its strength. This new stage is referred to as catabolism, the beginning and continuation of the aging process.

> "You can't help getting older, but you don't
> have to get old." —George Burns

The Aging Process by Body Part

Most people have experience with aging, either personally or through watching their parents or grandparents become elderly and, in some cases, frail. During aging, there are blatant signs, and then there are others that are subtle, less noticeable to the untrained eye. On the next page is a list of things that happen to the body as the years progress. By understanding the expected measurable signs of aging, we can take steps to slow the process and address specific areas of concern. This type of proactive approach will keep us all from waking up one day and wondering, "What happened?"

Part of the Body	Age of Decline	Functional and Physiological Changes
Brain	45	Decrease in mental reasoning, loss of focus, and trouble with memory. Interestingly, vocabulary does not decline, leaving many with undiagnosed brain changes. After the age of 20, the brain shrinks in size by 1% per year, but does so even faster when alcohol, smoking, or lack of sleep play a role.
Eyes	40	Eyesight is often the first sense to be affected by age. Difficulty reading in dim light due to aging pupils; loss of lens flexibility, making it harder to read things close up; yellowing lens, affecting color vision; and the development of cataracts are all age-related changes.
Ears	Varies by exposure to loud noises during life. Thirty percent of people over 65 have hearing loss.	Hearing loss, especially in higher tones, is common as we age. This is due to the loss of the tiny hairs within the ears that necessary for detecting sound waves. These hairs do not regrow, so most hearing loss is permanent. Balance is also affected by aging ears. The small bones within the ear that control our balance thicken with age, and can cause unsteadiness.
Skin	40 (and earlier in smokers and those with poor diets)	Changes in connective tissue in our skin cause loss of elasticity. There is a decrease in collagen, the substance that provides plumpness to the skin. Aging also slows the healing process and makes us more susceptible to bruising. The thinning epidermis (outer layer) reduces the insulation or padding that once made the skin appear youthful.

Part of the Body	Age of Decline	Functional and Physiological Changes
Kidneys	Varies with overall health conditions. For example, diabetics see a rapid decline in kidney function as they age.	Nephrons, which filter waste material from the blood, decrease in number as we age. The overall amount of kidney tissue also decreases, making the kidneys weaker. The blood vessels supplying each kidney can become hardened, causing a slower filtration. The aged bladder fails to empty completely, causing an increase in frequency of urinary tract infections.
Heart	35	Poor diet and exercise habits can lead to hardening of the arteries. Blockages, high blood pressure, and trouble pumping or filling can all cause problems. By the age of 50, the average heart muscle has contracted more than 2 billion times.
Lungs	After 20	Lung tissue decreases after the age of 20. Loss of elasticity and capacity also continues. Aging creates a greater risk of respiratory infection because the sensory receptors that keep pollutants from reaching the deep lung tissues become less effective. The amount of oxygen entering the blood from the air sacs decreases. At about 30 years of age, the rate of airflow through the airways slowly declines.
Pancreas	After 20	Decreased pancreatic fluid with age causes a decrease in the ability to breakdown carbohydrates, proteins, and lipids, which in turn slows metabolism. Over time, the pancreas produces less insulin, which increases the risk for diabetes mellitus.
Circulatory System	After 30	Stiffness in the small and large vessels decreases blood flow as we age. Also, decreased blood volume can create pooling in the legs. This can lead to decreased aerobic capacity, especially in those with sedentary lifestyles.

Part of the Body	Age of Decline	Functional and Physiological Changes
DNA	Varies with levels of stress, environmental factors, and nutrition.	Telomeres, the ends of chromosomes, begin to shorten. This inhibits the body's ability to heal itself. Like a wick on a candle, when the telomeres shorten completely, death is imminent.

While aging is a natural decline, many factors hasten the process. Often, these factors are completely preventable, but unfortunately many people overlook or disregard the warnings. Individuals should be able to enjoy each decade of life. The rate of aging should be slow and steady instead of quick and compounding.

Speed Aging

This book contains a wealth of information on many of the factors that speed the aging process, but this chapter wouldn't be complete without a list of items that are sure to put your aging into high gear. While genetics play a small role in what may lead to an early death, the majority of premature deaths are caused by personal lifestyle choices.

Micronutrient deficiencies. A poor diet can lead to deficiencies in the nutrients that are necessary for maintaining the body's homeostasis. Due to current soil conditions, it's hard to get the nutrients we need from food alone.

Increased body fat. A total body fat ratio above 25% for males and 32% for females is considered high risk. Elevated body fat is associated with heart disease, diabetes, stroke, sleep disorders, and even some cancers.

High stress levels. Stress is known to shorten telomeres and cause premature aging, so stress can negatively affect us even at the cellular level. Stress also causes weight gain, sleep disorders, and fatigue. Continued high levels of stress can take years off one's life.

Sedentary lifestyle. Exercise is essential to normal body function. A sedentary lifestyle leads to weight gain, diabetes, depression, and heart disease.

Sleep deprivation. The body needs at least 7.5 hours of sleep per night. Sleep is vital to the function of the heart, brain, and central nervous system as a whole. Lack of quality sleep can also cause weight gain, which leads to a number of other health problems. Losing 30 minutes of sleep each night may not seem like much, but it adds up to 15 hours lost each month, or 180 hours per year.

Environmental exposures. Pollutants can cause premature aging of the body as a whole. Once free radicals enter the body through exposure to pollutants, it's up to the immune system to clear them out. Even the strongest immune systems can't keep up with toxic environments.

Smoking. Cigarette smoke, either directly or secondhand, is the number one cause of early death in the United States. In the first month after quitting smoking, the lungs will begin to regenerate, but it will take 10 years to reverse the increased risk of cancer.

Alcohol. There is a reason that drinkers, especially those that drink heavily, have a prunish look about them. Alcohol inhibits the body's ability to absorb calcium, leaving the bones brittle and more likely to break. It is also considered a neurotoxin, causing deterioration in the frontal lobes of the brain. And about that prunish look: alcohol limits the body's ability to absorb and use amino acids, which are essential for a youthful appearance.

Who's Living the Longest?

Scientists have observed that certain populations, or subcultures, live an exceptionally long time. What may be perfect for one ethnicity with certain genetic traits may not be the same secret formula for another. It's important to understand that genetic makeup, on average, only accounts for one-third of the aging process. A long, healthy life depends far more on individual choice than genetic makeup. While these groups have many differences, they also have overlapping characteristics.

Okinawa, a remote Japanese island, has a population of one million, and 900 or more of them are centenarians. This is four times the number of those living in America. Unlike their North American counterparts, Okinawans have as many men as women seeing their tenth decade. Okinawans actually age the slowest of all of us on this planet, and at age 70, they are comparable in health to the average 50-year-old. This population seems to be almost immune to heart disease and certain cancers, even stomach cancer, which is usually most common among people of Japanese descent.

"Nobody grows old merely by living a number of years. We grow old by deserting our ideals. Years may wrinkle the skin, but to give up enthusiasm wrinkles the soul." —Samuel Ullman

Okinawans have a diet that is high in soy and tofu. This may explain why the centenarians in this part of the world have higher levels of DHEA, a steroid that is produced in the adrenal glands and is a precursor to hormones such as estrogen and testosterone. Their diet is also high in a wide range of fresh vegetable and fruits—all high in antioxidants. Known to clear the body of free radicals, antioxidants play an important role in overall health.

Sometimes it's not just what you eat, but how much you eat that counts. Even healthy food in excess can have bad effects. In Okinawa, they have a tradition of only eating until you are 80% full, or as they say, *hara hachi bu*. Typically, they consume 1,200 calories per day, compared to the average American who consumes as many as 3,400 calories—enough to feed three Okinawans.

In Ovodda, Sardinia (Italy), more than 6,300 miles from Okinawa, another nest of centenarians and super-centenarians (greater than 110) exist. With little to no soy, their diet is quite different, and lean meat is commonly eaten. They also avoid processed carbohydrates—what we usually refer to as "junk food." They eat high amounts of legumes and whole grains, with almost all of their nutritional options falling on the low side of the glycemic index. (See "Road Map 2: Glycemic Index" at the end of this chapter.)

Their diet is high in locally grown sun-ripened grapes. Nuts and olives also grow on their land and are readily available for consumption. In place of sugar, they use raw honey as a sweetener. Local honey has long been known to ward off allergies, and probably accounts for their strong immune systems.

The men of Sardinia are usually sheepherders and spend their days roaming rough terrain, getting quite a cardiovascular workout. The women, while not out in the fresh air as much as men, remain physically active doing work within their homes. For this population especially, good nutrition and plenty of exercise has really paid off.

A little closer to home, certain religious groups in America live longer than others. For example, Loma Linda, California, has a high population of Seventh-day Adventists, a group that lives a healthier lifestyle as dictated by their religion. Their vegetarian diet, as recommended by the Seventh-day Adventist Dietetic Association, consists of nine or more daily servings of vegetables and fruits and six servings of whole grains and legumes.

Cancer death rates for Seventh-day Adventists are 60% lower for men and 75% lower for women than the U.S. national average. Likewise, the rate of coronary heart disease is 66% lower for men and 98% lower for women as compared with others in the same geographical locations who are not Seventh-day Adventists. This religious group also encourages a healthy lifestyle with plenty of exercise, no alcohol, and no smoking—all things that promote longevity.

Much like the Seventh-day Adventists, the Church of Latter Day Saints, commonly referred to as Mormons, have an increase of longevity within their membership as compared with the general population. They, too, promote a healthy lifestyle free of alcohol and tobacco, but also include coffee and black teas on their list of no-nos. A recently completed 25-year study by researchers at the University of California, Los Angeles (UCLA) found that Mormon men live 10 years longer than non-Mormon men, and Mormon women live almost six years longer than non-Mormon women in the United States.

> "You are as young as your faith, as old as your doubt; as young as your self-confidence, as old as your fear; as young as your hope, as old as your despair." —Douglas MacArthur

The Mormon culture is strong in their faith, attending church at least once a week. Likewise, 52% of Mormons pray daily, compared with 58% of the population. Numerous studies have linked religious attendance and prayer to longevity, consistently showing that those who attend a place of worship least once a week live longer. Furthermore, the Mormon faith's strong emphasis on family and community makes nurturing one another a top priority. This strong fellowship lowers the stress and anxiety levels of its members.

The Mormon religion also emphasizes the importance of education, both religious and secular. Like many studies in the past, recent research conducted by the University of Wisconsin Population Health Institute and the Robert Wood Johnson Foundation found a strong link between education level and overall health. Mormons have a large number of educated members, with 54% of their men and 44% of their women in the United States having a higher education, compared to only a 27% national average. Good nutrition, daily prayer, healthy relationships, and higher education are all part of the equation, adding years to their lives.

Slowing the Process

Within the pages of this book, the focus is on slowing the aging process. If we learn to view aging as a syndrome, or a disease, then we can best plan the strategy for remission, or at least a slower decline. An all-encompassing approach to health and wellness will produce the best long-term results.

There is a great deal of information to be gleaned from the cultures that have mastered the aging process:

1. Eat a diet high in antioxidants to prevent cancer and inflammation.

2. Exercise regularly in an effort to keep your heart strong and your body mobile and flexible.

3. Use your brain continuously, whether it's reading or doing puzzles. Your brain needs to be exercised just like the muscles in your body.

4. Reduce stress. Find healthy ways to deal with the adversity in your life.

5. Expand your lungs with plenty of fresh air each and every day.

6. Avoid contaminants such as alcohol and tobacco.

7. Find a place of spiritual centeredness.

8. Make family a priority.

9. Help others. Volunteering is known to increase health and add years to your life.

10. Restrict calories, taking in only what your body actually needs. Avoid the all-you-can-eat buffets and make a continuous effort to manage portion size.

Even if you have been on the fast track to premature aging, it's never too late to improve your health. Take time to reflect on your attitude about aging and address your fears. Chances are that you will be able to take firm control over the situation and make steps today that will give you a brighter outlook for many, many tomorrows to come.

Highs and Lows—What Is the Glycemic Index?

The glycemic index (GI) is a scale used to rank foods based on how much they will raise your blood sugar levels. Using a range of 0–100, foods are given a number based on how they compare to straight glucose, which ranks as 100. When a food with a high GI is eaten, the body tries to normalize blood sugar levels by secreting insulin, the hormone that enables glucose to be absorbed into the cells where it is used for energy. Maintaining relatively stable blood sugar levels helps the body perform most efficiently. Research conducted at the Harvard School of Public Health found a strong relationship between high-glycemic diets and the development of heart disease and type 2 diabetes. Multiple other researchers have confirmed these findings.

Obesity is a growing problem (no pun intended), especially in the Western world. The foods we eat today are very different from those consumed a hundred years ago. When foods were being grown on site and taken straight to the table for consumption, they stayed in their purest form. Today, foods are stripped of many of their natural nutrients during processing and packaging. Over-processed food is digested rapidly, causing hunger pains to return quickly.

If the body takes in more glucose than it needs, that sugar will be stored as fat. This excess fat is usually found around the abdomen and is a precursor to a number of diseases known for speeding the aging process. Eating foods in their purest form, especially those with a low GI, will help prevent unnecessary glucose within the body and help maintain a healthy weight.

The Western diet is rich in high-glycemic foods, with more than 18% of the caloric intake being composed of sugar. White flour, which also has a high glycemic index, also accounts for another 18% of the average caloric intake. Nutritional choices make all the difference, and as you can see from the GI chart below, there is quite a contrast between a baked potato with a GI of 111 and hummus with a GI of only 6.

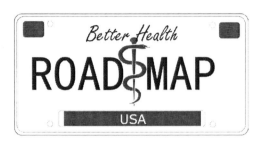

Low Glycemic Foods = 0–54 EAT THESE FOODS AS PART OF A DAILY DIET
Moderate Glycemic Foods = 55–69 EAT SPARINGLY or WITH CAUTION
High Glycemic Foods = 70 or Greater STOP or TRY TO AVOID

GRAINS	GLYCEMIC INDEX (glucose = 100)
Pearled barley	28
Whole wheat kernels	30
Converted, white rice (Uncle Ben's®)	38
Bulgur	48
Brown rice	50
Quinoa	53
Sweet corn on the cob	60
Couscous	65
Quick cooking white rice	67
White rice	89

PASTA AND NOODLES	GLYCEMIC INDEX (glucose = 100)
Fettucini, average	32
Spaghetti, whole wheat, boiled, average	42
Spaghetti, white, boiled, average	46
Macaroni, average	47
Spaghetti, white, boiled 20 min, average	58
Macaroni and cheese (Kraft®)	64

FRUITS	GLYCEMIC INDEX (glucose = 100)
Prunes	15
Grapefruit	25
Prunes, pitted	29
Pear	38
Apple	39
Orange	40
Peach	42
Pear, canned in pear juice	43
Peach, canned in light syrup	52
Grapes	59
Banana, ripe	62
Raisins	64
Watermelon	72
Dates	103

BEANS AND NUTS	GLYCEMIC INDEX (glucose = 100)
Almonds	0
Peanuts	7
Chickpeas	10
Walnuts	15
Soy beans	15
Cashews, salted	27
Kidney beans	29
Lentils	29
Black beans	30
Navy beans	31
Black-eyed peas	33
Baked beans	40

SNACK FOODS	GLYCEMIC INDEX (glucose = 100)
Hummus (chickpea salad dip)	6
M & M's®, peanut	33
Corn chips, plain, salted, average	42
Potato chips, average	56
Snickers bar®	51
Microwave popcorn, plain, average	55
Fruit Roll-Ups®	99

BREAKFAST CEREALS	GLYCEMIC INDEX (glucose = 100)
All-Bran™	55
Oatmeal	55
Raisin Bran™ (Kellogg's)	61
Cream of Wheat™ (Nabisco)	66
Muesli, average	66
Special K™ (Kellogg's)	69
Cream of Wheat™, Instant (Nabisco)	74
Grape-Nuts™	75
Corn Pops™	80
Puffed wheat	80
Instant oatmeal	83
Rice Chex™	89
Corn Flakes™	93

COOKIES AND CRACKERS	GLYCEMIC INDEX (glucose = 100)
Shortbread	64
Rye crisps, average	64
Wheat Thins®	67
Graham crackers	74
Soda crackers	74
Vanilla wafers	77
Rice cakes	80
Rice cakes, average	82
Pretzels, oven-baked	83

VEGETABLES	GLYCEMIC INDEX (glucose = 100)
Spinach, raw	0
Broccoli	15
Carrots	35
Green peas	51
Parsnips	52
Yam	54
Beets	64
Sweet potato	70
Boiled white potato	82
Instant mashed potato	87
Baked russet potato	111

BAKERY PRODUCTS AND BREADS	GLYCEMIC INDEX (glucose = 100)
Wheat tortilla	30
Coarse barley bread, 75%-80% kernels, average	34
Vanilla cake made from packet mix with vanilla frosting (Betty Crocker™)	42
Sponge cake, plain	46
Banana cake, made with sugar	47
Corn tortilla	52
Pumpernickel bread	56
Hamburger bun	61
Pita bread, white	68
White bread	71
Whole wheat bread	71
White bagel	72
Kaiser roll	73
Wonder™ bread, average	73
Waffles, Aunt Jemima™	76
Baguette, white, plain	95

SWEETENERS	GLYCEMIC INDEX (glucose = 100)
Agave syrup	15
Fructose	22
Honey, raw	30
Sugar cane juice	43
Maple syrup	54
Honey, average	61
High-fructose corn syrup	62
Brown sugar	64
Sucrose (table sugar)	65

DAIRY PRODUCTS AND ALTERNATIVES	GLYCEMIC INDEX (glucose = 100)
Yogurt , plain	14
Milk, skim	32
Reduced-fat yogurt with fruit, average	33
Ice cream, premium	38
Milk, full fat	41
Ice cream, regular	57

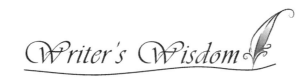
Writer's Wisdom

JUST YOU AND THE OPEN ROAD

When I'm not in a suit and tie, I'm on my Harley. I recently took a much needed road trip: 2 countries, 12 states, and 3,255 miles—all solo. I prepared for my journey by making sure both the bike and I were in good shape. New tires, enough rest, all the right gear to make the trip. I knew the general direction of where I wanted to go but didn't map out a specific route. The goal was to end up back at the starting point nine days later. While some stops were on the map, the most inspiring ones were those that were off the beaten path.

Just like my journey on the bike, a journey to better health is all about the preparation and the paths you take. There will be challenges along the way, but with preparation and openness to change, you can meet and overcome each challenge with strength and courage. Just as the old cliché states: "Life is a journey, not a destination."

If you think of your body as the vehicle of life, you must take good care of it. It needs good fuel, plenty of road time (exercise), necessary maintenance, and frequent inspections. Bumps will happen. Storms will come...some you will have to push through, others you just have to wait out. However, if you are well prepared, these too will come to pass. By the way, it is always a good idea to have something to read while waiting (this book is a good choice).

Along this journey of life you will make great friends, find love, lose it, and find it again, and say hello and good-bye to loved ones. But if you are fortunate, the trip will end where it began, with many, many, good memories in between.

—J. Mark Anderson, MD

CHAPTER THREE

BECOMING THE RULE, NOT THE EXCEPTION

Why we are living longer

"I look to the future because that's where I'm going
to spend the rest of my life." —George Burns

I am sure you remember the day when turning 100 years old was quite the accomplishment, when part of the fun of watching the morning news was to see some very aged person from somewhere across the country blowing out 100 candles. Today, there are over 80,000 Americans who are living as centenarians, compared to just over 37,000 in 1990, and the number is expected to grow exponentially. In countries with high life expectancy rates, the life span average is going up by six hours per day. That's the same as 91 days per year, or roughly two and a half years per decade.

What Is Life Expectancy?

Whenever you hear the term "life expectancy," it refers to the average life expectancy of someone born that year. When calculating life expectancy, the Centers for Disease Control and Prevention (CDC) takes into account death from childhood diseases, teen car accidents, death during childbirth for both the mother and child, and so on. Therefore, the real life expectancy is fluid and changes as we age. Each time we hit a milestone, our life expectancy goes up. If you are alive at age 65, your life expectancy goes up by several years because you have already survived all types of potential death traps. If you make it to 75, your life expectancy continues to increase. By age 100, your likelihood of death is 50/50 each year going forward.

Life expectancy is changing, and according to Dr. James Vaupel, the head of Duke University's Center on the Demography of Aging, most children born after the year 2000 will live to see their 100th birthday. Of course, this leads to a number of questions about public policy, healthcare, and the future landscape of the human race. With each passing month adding three months to the average life expectancy, necessary changes will be coming fast and furious.

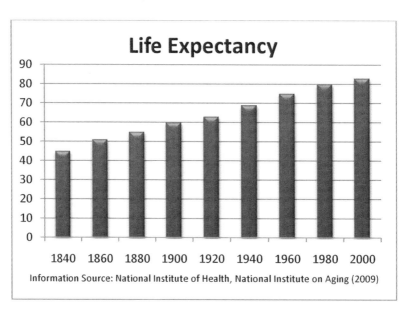

Information Source: National Institute of Health, National Institute on Aging (2009)

How We Got Here

These days, you can look at someone in their 40s and appreciate the amount of life ahead of them. Just 100 years ago, reaching age 50 would have been quite the accomplishment. There have been 10 great achievements in the 20th century that extended life and brought us to where we are today. While many of these are simply routine and taken for granted, these milestones changed mankind and its future forever.

1. Vaccinations and Immunizations

While most of us can't imagine burying our own child, it was commonplace for families in the 1800s, with most families losing at least one if not more of their children. Without immunizations, illnesses like the flu claimed millions of lives. According to statistics, 50 million people died in the influenza epidemic of 1918. This is more than the number of people killed in the entire First World War. This number becomes especially staggering when compared with the current annual flu deaths, which number about 36,000 in the United States.

2. Seatbelts and Safer Vehicles

It is no secret that seatbelts, car seats, and airbags save lives. Motor vehicle travel has increased tenfold since the 1920s, but despite this increase, less people are dying on roads than ever before. In the 1920s, the CDC states that the annual motor vehicle death rate was 18 deaths per every 100 million miles driven. By the late 1990s, this number had dropped to 1.7 deaths per every 100 million miles driven. This 90% decrease speaks to the inestimable improvements in vehicle safety that took place in the 20th century. As the automobile industry continually implements newer, more advanced safety measure, the vehicle-related death rate is expected to continue to decline.

3. Improvement in Working Conditions

In the past, common laborers put their lives in the hands of their employer each day. Factories and mines were beset with potential hazards at every turn. In 1907, more than 500 steelworkers died in just one U.S. state; fast forward 100 years to 2007 in which there were only 17 steelworker deaths in the entire nation.

4. Modern Plumbing

An amenity that is often taken for granted, modern plumbing directly relates to the health of a society. While waste-borne diseases such as cholera are still a leading cause of death in developing nations, they no longer ravage the Western world to the extent that they once did. Wherever modern plumbing is implemented, life expectancy is drastically extended.

5. Cardiovascular Death Reduction

According to the CDC, cardiovascular disease accounts for over one-third of deaths in the United States. Despite this, more people are surviving heart attacks and strokes, a trend attributed to improvements in healthcare over the last decade. Today, many people walk away from a heart attack or stroke and partially or completely recover—something unheard of a century ago when cardiovascular events meant certain death.

6. FDA and Food Safety

In 1906, Upton Sinclair published his novel *The Jungle,* a groundbreaking critique of the hugely problematic meatpacking industry. It is no coincidence that this is the same year in which the Food and Drug Administration's (FDA's) modern regulatory purpose was established, through the passage of the Pure Food and Drugs Act. Regulatory action and heightened public awareness of sanitary food conditions greatly reduced the chances of food-borne illnesses. As the original consumer protection agency in the United States, the FDA continues to enact policy and regulate medicine and food with the health of our country as its primary goal.

7. Improvements in Childbirth

As late as the early 1900s, childbirth was still a relatively high-risk endeavor. For every 1,000 live births, six to nine women died of complications, and 100 infants, or 10%, did not live to see their first birthday. A flurry of 20th-century improvements in everything from disease monitoring to maternal health to clinical medicine have greatly improved the risk factor of childbirth. By 1997, mortality rates had declined by over 90%, with 7.2 infant deaths per 1,000 live births and less than 0.1% maternal deaths. The CDC describes this as the most significant decrease in mortality rates during the 20th century.

8. Birth Control

Imagine that every time you had sex with your spouse you would risk bringing another life into this world. Before birth control, this was the reality faced by husbands and wives. Of course, this risk was especially grave for women, as pregnancy required a nearly year-long dedication to carrying the child. Since avoiding sex was out of the question, families were generally much larger in size, increasing the risk of death from childbirth complications.

9. Improved Dental Care

In the past, bad teeth wasn't just unattractive, it was downright deadly. One of the best public health initiatives was to fluoridate the drinking water. Not only did this policy prevent cavities that could potentially lead to raging infections, it undoubtedly improved mortality rates in other ways. We now know there is a link between heart disease and poor dental hygiene. As research continues, scientists are finding out just how interconnected seemingly unrelated health issues really are.

10. Tobacco Reduction

It may be difficult to appreciate how widely accepted cigarette smoking was during most of the 20th century, and how little awareness people had of the dangers of smoking. However, until the U.S. Surgeon General's 1964 statement, public knowledge about the hazardous effects of smoking cigarettes was minimal at best. The official 1964 statement, warning that "cigarette smoking is a health hazard of sufficient importance to warrant appropriate remedial action," was the first step in a long procession of policy and scientific efforts to raise public knowledge and reduce tobacco consumption. While work remains to be done, past decades have shown a decline in smoking of at least 50%. Between the harms inflicted on the smoker and the effects of long-term exposure to secondhand smoke, this much needed change has led to a healthier population.

Today, people are living longer because of these achievements in public health. However, when it comes to the spike in life expectancy, the story is just beginning. Scientific discovery, specifically at the genetic level, is giving us insight into the processes of aging. As we begin to understand not just the genetic risks but how to protect our DNA from harmful mutations, longevity will become the rule, not the exception.

"What more powerful form of study of mankind could there be
than to read our own instruction book?" —Francis S. Collins

What the Future Holds

The Human Genome Project (HGP), completed in 2003, was a 13-year project coordinated by the U.S. Department of Energy and the National Institutes of Health. This collaboration of scientists from different nations working to understand the human body was more than a scientific feat: it was a global triumph. It affirmed a belief in our underlying humanity, a humanity that transcends political borders.

Through the HGP, the tens of thousands of genes that comprise a human have been mapped out and studied. This understanding of what makes us who we are paves the way for new discoveries that will shape our health and wellness for the rest of time. Our DNA holds the answers to eliminating disease and slowing the aging process. In short, it holds the key to our lengthening future.

Once the human genome was mapped out, Dr. George Church, a Harvard professor and leading scientist in genomics, began work on the Personal Genome Project (PGP). Volunteers from all over the world have submitted their DNA to help propel forward the mapping and understanding of our genetic makeup. Dr. Church, interestingly enough, was the first to volunteer his DNA for mapping. We, the authors, recently had our DNA sequenced as well through the 23andMe project. Just as George Church saw a vision of how his own personal contribution of DNA could further mankind, we as leaders in proactive and preventative medicine also felt it was our duty. The results were fascinating. Having a personal road map to our bodies allows us to understand our genetic risk factors and devise a plan of action. Knowledge of one's body on a cellular level provides a greater understanding of mortality risks, an invaluable insight that shapes future choices. Having our DNA sequenced made us keenly cognizant of the importance of our daily lifestyle choices.

In the future, many medications will be tailor-made to the specific needs of your DNA. This is referred to as pharmacogenomics, and it is being used right now with cancer treatments. Moving forward, our own DNA will be able to identify which medications, or class of drugs, will most benefit our individual bodies. Physicians are left with many choices when writing a patient's prescription; this will help narrow their decisions.

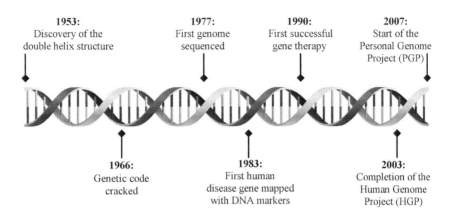

1953:
Discovery of the
double helix structure

1977:
First genome
sequenced

1990:
First successful
gene therapy

2007:
Start of the
Personal Genome
Project (PGP)

1966:
Genetic code
cracked

1983:
First human
disease gene mapped
with DNA markers

2003:
Completion of the
Human Genome
Project (HGP)

The entire landscape of the pharmaceutical world is changing. As it continues to change, its greatest challenge may not be the science, but the FDA, which was not set up to review individualized medications, but rather to review mass-produced drugs and their effectiveness and safety on the population as a whole. These kinds of challenges will force the FDA to enlist leaders in the field of pharmacogenomics as consultants.

Dr. Aubrey De Grey, a biomedical gerontologist, is dedicated to finding ways for people to stay healthier longer. A man ahead of his time, he has been making predictions about extended life long before it was popular to do so. His view, which is shared by many medical doctors involved with the science of aging, is that patients will stop going to the doctor for illness, and instead will go for maintenance visits that may include things like gene therapy, immune stimulation, stem cell therapy, or even things that haven't yet been discovered.

Aging is a disease, but until we treat it as one, our bodies will continue to break down on the cellular level, causing the diseases that now end life so prematurely. Dr. De Grey believes that in the next two decades, the first person to reach their 1,000th birthday will be born. To most people, this may sound like a bit of a stretch, but only time will tell. As Dr. Anderson observes in the introduction, Da Vinci and other visionaries of his day were the fuel that sparked the Italian Renaissance. As medicine embarks on a journey of cellular and genetic discovery, who are we to thwart the insights of a man so highly experienced and dedicated to his field of study?

Scientists are estimating that the children born today may very well reach their

150th birthdays. This generation will not just live longer, but healthier, so don't expect them to spend their last 50 years in a nursing home. Throughout the journey of life, human interests are constantly evolving in response to changing bodies and new experiences. As lifespan increases, expect to see not just second careers, but third and fourth ones.

Just as it's hard for us to look back to a time when the average life span was 60 years of age, our children and their children will soon find it hard to believe that people died in their 80s and 90s. Right now, we have the technology and medical advancements to detect disease in the earliest stages, slowing the aging process. Each person has choices to make regarding their health. They can either go from one day to the next accepting the status quo, or take charge of their future. Being proactive will make a significant difference in not only how long they live, but how well they live out those later years. With the exception of some circumstances, personal choices will determine if the last memories are those of four walls and a wheelchair, or memorable vacations and full mobility.

"We are here to celebrate the completion of the first survey of the entire human genome. Without a doubt, this is the most important, most wondrous map ever produced by human kind." —President Bill Clinton (*from White House press conference broadcast on the day of the publication of the first draft of the human genome*)

CHAPTER FOUR

GAINING LATITUDE WITH THE RIGHT ATTITUDE

The science behind being happy

"True happiness is...to enjoy the present, without anxious dependence upon the future." —Lucius Annaeus Seneca

Most health and wellness books will advise you on what to eat, how to exercise, when to see the doctor, and all the usual rhetoric on how to stay healthy, but few address the importance of attitude. At its core, health begins with the individual: the amount of stress they allow into their world and how they respond to adversity. The age-old adage teaches us: What you think, you will become. If you tell yourself you are old and sick, eventually your body will respond to what it's being told. According to a compilation of over 30 studies, being happy and having a good attitude can add 7.5–10 years to your life. Positive thinking could be the difference between seeing that grandchild or great-grandchild, or not.

Everyone will face adversity in life, whether it's the death of a loved one, divorce, disappointment, or unexpected health issues. Waiting until a time of crisis to learn coping skills is like going out to buy a fire extinguisher while the house is burning down. The body will not have backup defenses to deal with its physiological changes amidst a disaster unless it's trained to do so. Teach yourself to be content regardless of your circumstances and you will be ready to tackle challenges as they arise. You can actually train your body to self-regulate in stressful situations, but this will take time.

Happiness is like a bank account, with positive experiences and emotions being the deposits and negative ones being the withdrawals. This very concept has intrigued researchers and led them to develop the "happiness formula." Dr. Barbara Fredrickson, the principal investigator at the University of North Carolina Positive Emotions and Psychology Lab, has unveiled a link between positive emotions and physical health. The formula for maintaining health and resisting the ill effects of stress and adversity occurs in a 3:1 ratio, meaning you need three positive emotions to every negative one. Maintaining this ratio may take a little work on your part, but just like anything else in life, the most beneficial things take effort.

*INSTANT*INSIGHT   Clothing can say a great deal about a person's state of mind. A recent study showed a strong correlation between a woman's outfit and her mood. Woman who were sad or depressed were more likely to wear loose clothing, such as sweats or baggy tops. Those who dressed up in a nice outfit and put effort into their appearance had more positive emotions. So, next time you need a boost, start in the closet.

So, why are some people just grumpy or mean? Are they born that way? Well, yes and no. After 20 years of research, Dr. Sonja Lyubomirsky, Professor at the University of California, Riverside, found that 50% of one's attitude is attributed to genes, 40% to intentional activities, and 10% to life circumstances such as socioeconomic class, marital status, or health. Some people are born with a smile on their face and others with a chip on their shoulder. The latter need to work extra hard to control their intentional activities and circumstances, or they will destine themselves to a life of disappointment and misery. Along with such negative emotions comes poor health. Research has told us time and time again that at the core of a long and healthy life is a perpetual smile.

The best way to control your attitude is to first control your thoughts and your tongue. Sarcasm and gossip need to be banished from your life because nothing good evolves from either one. Every person and every circumstance has a positive aspect, but sometimes you just have to look deeper to find it. If you focus on the good, you will learn to recognize it more easily and gain a better sense of gratitude in your life. It's an exercise that will strengthen your ability to be positive and will benefit your health and the health of your family. When negative experiences come your way, and they will from time to time, learn how to control your reaction. How you react to negativity will determine how long those feelings linger and the overall impact they have on your health. You may not be able to change your circumstances, but you can keep your circumstances from changing you.

Rising Above It All

While there are thousands, if not millions, of stories of inspiration, one of our favorite examples of overcoming adversity comes from someone who was born over 200 years ago, back when modern conveniences and modern healthcare were not available. John Rowe Moyle left his home in England and traveled to Salt Lake City because of his religious convictions. Most of his journey was hard labor, as he pushed a hand cart through miles of treacherous conditions. He settled into a small town a ways from Salt Lake. Shortly after his arrival, he was asked to help build the Salt Lake Temple by sharing his skills as an accomplished stone cutter. Honored to do this work, he left home on Mondays at two o'clock in the morning to walk six hours to the building site, and left work on Fridays at five o'clock to arrive back home by midnight. This went on for years. He was content with his life, doing what he loved for a cause he believed in. I am sure you have all been there at some point, and can relate to his feeling of happy exhaustion.

> "There is a fountain of youth: it is your mind, your talents, the creativity you bring to your life and the lives of people you love. When you learn to tap this source, you will truly have defeated age." —Sophia Loren

One weekend, while doing the necessary chores on the home front, the unthinkable happened. Moyle was kicked in the leg by his milk cow and suffered a compound fracture, the type that leaves the bone sticking out through the skin. Without the medical resources we have today, his future was almost certain death. Even if he didn't bleed to death, infection should have taken his life. His friends and family did what they had to do. Moyle was strapped to a door which had been taken off its hinges. His leg was then amputated with a bucksaw, a far cry from today's clinical standards. The likelihood of such a crude surgery being a success without terminal infection was unheard of. Many in his circumstances would have chosen to just give up. At that point, Moyle had a choice to make. And he did.

He kept a positive attitude and set a goal to return to work in Salt Lake City. He carved his own wooden leg and even added a fake joint that served as an ankle, something that had not been done before. His ingenuity and optimism were at the very center of his healing process. He taught himself how to walk again and built up the strength and endurance to make his 22-mile trek back to the temple to continue the work he loved so much.

Moyle even taught himself how to climb the towering scaffolding so that he could inscribe the message "Holiness to the Lord" that over a 100 years later can still be seen be seen for miles around. The message has been read by people from all walks of life. His attitude directly affected his health and his future, and should be a lesson to all of us, regardless of our struggles. Because Moyle didn't give up, he was able to leave his mark on the world long after he faced his biggest trial. When you are having a bad day or want to give up, remember the courage and strength that this man had, and let it serve as a reminder to you to keep going. Sometimes the trials we face are a precursor to our most surprising victories.

> "A healthy attitude is contagious, but don't wait to catch it from others. Be a carrier." —Tom Stoppard

Self-regulation plays a large role in managing emotional vitality. Learning how to control the very impulses that lead to stressful situations can prevent many of those situations from ever developing. For example, risky behaviors such as unsafe sex, overeating, or a sedentary lifestyle will lead to poor health and unnecessary anxiety, while a healthy diet and exercise will have a positive effect on the body and one's overall happiness. These are the things that make up the 40% intentional activities that can be attributed to one's attitude discussed earlier in this chapter.

So, let's go over what happens to the body physiologically during times of stress and also during times of happiness. Once you understand the basic health principles behind happiness, then finding the road to enduring happiness will hopefully become your first quest.

Stress Versus Happiness

Physiological changes during times of *enduring stress* include:

Increased heart rate (anxiety)

Increased blood pressure (increased risk for stroke)

Surges of cortisol and adrenaline (weight gain)

Decreased digestion (heartburn)

Decreased cognitive function (stupidity)

Changes in brain chemicals, especially the release of norepinephrine (depression)

Weakened immune system due to an inflammatory response (illness)

Neuroendocrine and immune dysfunction (increased risk of cancer)

Muscle cramps and spasm (pain)

Physiological changes during times of happiness include:

Lower and more stable blood pressure readings

Release of serotonin, the "feel good" hormone

Increased ability to maintain a healthy weight

Increased sense of smell and taste

Improved immunity due to increased T cells, a type of white blood cell

Decreased risk of cancer

Decreased risk of heart disease

Increased ability to recovery from illness

Increased tolerance to pain

Basically, you have a choice to make: You can settle for being prone to anxiety, weight gain, or illness, or you can learn to be grateful, no matter what your circumstances are. Gratitude leads to contentment with one's circumstances and, ultimately, happiness, which in turn has an abundance of health benefits. The goal is not only to live longer, but to live a long and satisfying life.

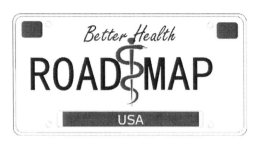

Satisfaction With Life Scale (SWLS)

Below are five statements that you may agree or disagree with. Using the 1–7 scale below,[1] indicate your agreement with each item by placing the appropriate number on the line preceding that item. Please be open and honest with your responses.

7—Strongly agree

6—Agree

5—Slightly agree

4—Neither agree nor disagree

3—Slightly disagree

2—Disagree

1—Strongly disagree

____ In most ways, my life is close to my ideal.

____ The conditions of my life are excellent.

____ I am satisfied with my life.

____ So far, I have gotten the important things I want in life.

____ If I could live my life over, I would change almost nothing.

Now add up your responses, and see where you fall in the ratings below:

31–35 Extremely satisfied

26–30 Satisfied

21–25 Slightly satisfied

20   Neutral

15–19 Slightly dissatisfied

10–14 Dissatisfied

5–9   Extremely dissatisfied

---

[1] Authors of the SWLS: Ed Diener, Robert A. Emmons, Randy J. Larsen, and Sharon Griffin, as noted in the 1985 article in the *Journal of Personality Assessment*.

When stressed and unhappy, messages taken in by the senses can't properly make it to the brain, causing a feeling of numbness. If you find yourself reading this chapter and thinking you don't have the first clue on how to "get happy," then start by taking baby steps in the right direction. First, turn off the television and go for a walk outside or visit a museum; this will help turn your senses back on and help you live in the moment. Do not take your cell phone or other electronic distractions. Second, take time to contemplate and appreciate the things in your life. It's easy to be so busy that one day runs into the next—until soon, a whole month, if not year, has passed by. If we don't take time to appreciate the details of each day, our whole lives will seem but a fleeting moment reminiscent of deadlines and anxiety. Last, spend time with friends and family each week. Don't wait for holidays or those times that you gather together out of obligation. Isn't it ironic that funerals are often the most attended family gatherings? Instead of mourning those missed opportunities, find meaningful ways to share moments together through volunteer projects or planned outings. A Harvard Medical School study found that you can catch happiness because the more social connections you have, the more likely you are to be happy. For the record, "social media" connections do not count.

If you don't own a pet, research says you should. Pets have been shown to ward off depression by elevating levels of serotonin and dopamine, which signal pleasure and calmness to the brain. Cortisol, the hormone that is released during stress, causing havoc on the body, is much lower in pet owners. In 1980, a Public Health report showed that pet owners who suffered a heart attack were 28% more likely to survive, compared with those without four-legged friends. Pet owners generally are more likely to get exercise, be less depressed, and show unconditional love toward others.

There are a number of medical conditions that can cause feelings of depression or unhappiness. The "happiness" versus "healthiness" dilemma is a chicken-and-egg scenario. If you aren't happy, you can't reach optimal health, and if you aren't healthy, it's hard, and sometimes medically impossible, to be inherently happy.

Of course, there are many health concerns that could lead to feelings of depression or anxiety. Be sure to give your physician a clear picture of your overall health, both physical and emotional. A complete physical exam that looks at sex hormone levels, thyroid function, inflammation, and organ function is essential to understanding the bigger picture of your well-being. Optimal health is achieved by first understanding your current health status and then taking steps to improve it.

As discussed in Chapter 7, micronutrient deficiencies are common and can lead to symptoms such as depression, eventually causing breakdown within the organ systems of the body. Be sure to review that chapter thoroughly, especially if you are experiencing symptoms of depression or lack of motivation. Too often, the answer is to prescribe medication to cover the symptoms instead of finding the root cause of the problem. Be proactive when talking with your physician about your emotional health concerns by requesting a complete physical, including comprehensive laboratory testing prior to being placed on mood-altering medications.

Happiness should be a goal for every individual. Smiling is as important to life as eating and breathing, and needs to be viewed that way. Take time each and every day to laugh and enjoy life. Don't just pursue happiness—create it!

Smile Styles

Guillaume Duchenne, a French physician and early researcher in the field of what is now known as neurology, studied the smile in the mid-19th century. He identified two distinct smile types. The most expressive type of smile, now known as the Duchenne smile, involves contracting the zygomatic major muscle, raising the corners of the mouth, and the orbicularis oculi muscle, raising the cheeks and creating wrinkles around the eyes. A non-Duchenne smile involves only the zygomatic major muscle, so the cheeks and eyes are not involved. Duchenne and other researchers believe that the Duchenne smile is the only one associated with positive emotion, making it the true sign of happiness.

In 2005, Drs. Ernest Abel and Michael Kruger from Wayne State University in Detroit, Michigan, reported a retrospective study on smiles and longevity. They reviewed photographs of the 1952 season of Major League baseball players, rating their expressions according to the following categories: no smile, a non-Duchenne smile, and a Duchenne Smile. Then they focused on the 150 players who had passed away as of June 2009. The players with no smile lived for an average of 72 years. Those who had a non-Duchenne smile lived to be about 75 years. Players who displayed a genuine Duchenne smile lived to about 80 years. Whoever said laughter is the best medicine wasn't very far off. This study just goes to show that a positive demeanor really can make a difference between life and death.

MARY LAUFFER, 95 YEARS YOUNG, ANNAPOLIS, MARYLAND

Lifetime golfer and National Senior Games Gold Medalist (2011; Personal Best profile at www.NSGA.com). "It's terrible to see people that are obese—they don't exercise and their eating habits are dreadful. They don't understand what they're doing to their bodies. I exercise and walk all the time—you just have to. I'm busy with a 50-up community here, and they are very active. Of course I play golf when the weather is good. Nutrition has become important, too. I'm fortunate that I have been able to stay healthy and keep doing what I'm doing."

CHAPTER FIVE

FIVE BIG KILLERS

Heart disease, diabetes, cancer, infection, and stress

"If you ask what is the single most important key to longevity,
I would have to say it is avoiding worry, stress and tension. And
if you didn't ask me, I'd still have to say it." —George Burns

The human body is multifaceted, and everything needs to be in proper working order. Much like a Swiss watch, one small thing out of place can impact the entire system, even affecting how long it will tick. If you don't want to clock out early, then be sure the intricacies of your body are functioning at full capacity and in harmony.

Although there are many ways to die, some deaths are more common than others. If the population is educated in the risks that lead to early death *and* they take responsibility for their own health, the statistics on mortality provided by the CDC could look very different.

This chapter provides an educational outline of the leading causes of death, and offers tips on how to make healthier choices. As mentioned in our chapter on personal responsibility, living to one 100 years, or even close to that number, takes dedication and vigilance. Good health starts with education and ends with ongoing due diligence.

Heart Disease

The American Heart Association estimates that every 25 seconds, an American will have a coronary event, and approximately every minute, someone will die of one. That means 60 deaths per hour, 1,440 deaths per day, and 525,600 deaths per year. It is estimated that 13 million Americans have some form of heart disease, making it the number one cause of death for both men and women in the United States. Heart disease is often a self-inflicted tragedy, because most of the deaths could have been prevented by making consistently healthier choices. A nutritious diet, regular exercise, and a yearly physical examination are the cure to America's top health problem.

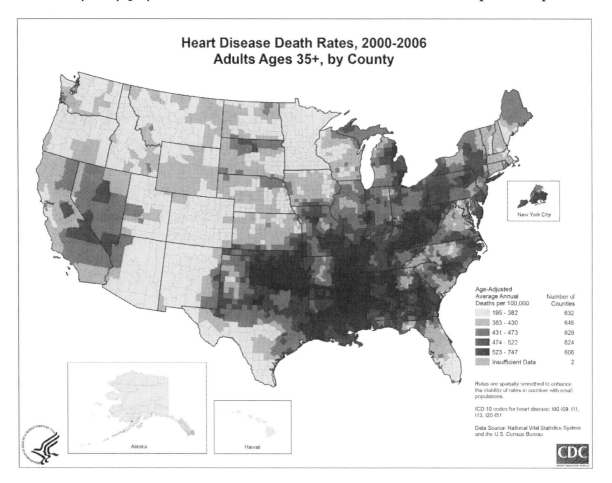

Unfortunately, obesity has become a major issue in the United States. This is especially concerning for the youth, who are more obese than at any other time in history. Childhood obesity is a risk factor for early death. Increases in body fat percentage, a sedentary lifestyle, and a proclivity for other unhealthy habits such as smoking have led to 33.5% of adults age 20 years and older having hypertension.

High blood pressure is no longer a problem just for middle-aged, pot-bellied men. It now infiltrates our society at a much younger age, and does not discriminate based on gender or ethnicity. The National Heart, Lung, and Blood Institute (NHLBI) has changed the parameters for hypertension to match new information we have on the risks associated with high blood pressure.

<u>KNOW YOUR NUMBERS:</u>

Normal blood pressure:

Less than 120 systolic (top number) and less than 80 diastolic (bottom number)

Prehypertension:

120–139 systolic and 80–89 diastolic

High blood pressure:

140 systolic and 90 or greater diastolic

Blockages and narrowing within the coronary arteries, also known as athero-sclerosis, are caused by the collection of fatty materials or plaque on the lining of the arteries. Most people think that heart attacks happen when an artery becomes completely blocked, but a person with just a 50% blockage could have a fatal heart attack. The risk of complete obstruction comes from the plaque rupturing and forming a clot. This is how people who pass a general checkup can drop dead the next day. Instead of a quick exam, it takes a compilation of tests to determine a patient's actual risk. Together, a good healthcare provider and compliant patient can keep those risks from developing into a life-threatening emergency.

There is now advanced testing that can determine the best plan of action for treating and preventing heart disease. For many years, doctors relied solely on the total cholesterol number. It wasn't until later that the total number was broken down into good (HDL) and bad (LDL) cholesterol. Now, new technology allows us to view particle size and subcategories of cholesterol. This data has demystified the phenomenon of patients with cholesterol levels of 250 dropping dead, while others with levels of 400 living long and virtually healthy lives. While it can be complicated to explain all the intricate details, the most significant data lies in the particle size. If a person has an LDL particle size that is Pattern A, he or she is less likely to develop life-threatening blockages because the LDL is large and buoyant, flowing through the arteries without attaching. Unfortunately, Pattern B–size particles of LDL are more likely to dig into the walls of the arteries, stick together, and form a blockage because they are small and dense.

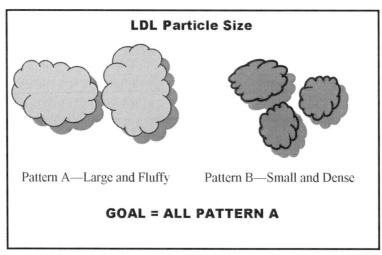

The heart disease problem is enormous in our society, and big steps need to be taken to get it under control. This is not something that can be fixed with a new healthcare system, better insurance, or stricter policies. Instead, each person needs to take personal responsibility and work toward a healthier self. Education is the only way to empower people to make changes. We feel strongly that if people have a full understanding of what heart disease is, what it does to the body, and how to prevent it, many lives could be spared.

KNOW YOUR RISKS: Heart Disease

___ High cholesterol or triglycerides

___ Pattern B LDL particle size

___ High blood pressure (baseline greater than 120/80)

___ Diabetes or pre-diabetes

___ Smoker or exposed to secondhand smoke

___ Lack of physical activity and a regular exercise routine

___ Waist size greater than 40 inches for men or greater than 35 inches for women

___ Diet that contains fewer than five to seven servings of fresh fruits or vegetables each day

___ High levels of stress at home or work

___ Strong family history of heart disease

___ Sleep deprivation (sleeping less than seven and a half hours per night, or having interrupted sleep cycles)

SAVE YOURSELF:

___ Exercise at least three times a week for 30 minutes each time
___ Eat no more than four ounces of red meat a day
___ Eat five to seven servings of *fresh* fruits and vegetables per day
___ Do not smoke or expose yourself to secondhand smoke
___ Keep your weight and waist size down
___ Decrease stress levels through exercise, yoga, reading, or journaling
___ Get a yearly physical exam, including the tests listed below

DIAGNOSTIC MUST-HAVES:

___ Advanced lipid panel, including particle size
___ Cardio C-reactive protein
___ Stress test (VO2Max stress test is even better—see Chapter 6)
___ Calcium score of the coronary arteries
___ Carotid doppler (screening for stroke risk)

Type 2 Diabetes

While there are two types of diabetes, for the sake of this chapter we will be discussing adult onset diabetes, also referred to as type 2, which is the most common form. Glucose is important for the body because it offers energy for muscle, fat, and the liver. When we eat, the sugar known as glucose enters the bloodstream and is delivered to the places that need it for energy. The glucose is not able to make it to the other parts of the body without something called insulin, which is produced in the pancreas. When a person has diabetes, the cells do not respond normally to insulin and the glucose remains in the bloodstream.

With 25.8 million children and adults suffering from diabetes, or 8.3% of the American population, this disease is at a record high. It is the seventh leading cause of death in our country. Diabetes is costing the country and individuals a fortune, with over $174 billion a year going to the care of known diabetics, and even more money going to treat the complications of those who are not diagnosed. According to a 2011 study out of Cambridge University in Britain, having diabetes shortens life by an average of six years. Of course, it goes without saying that diabetes affects the quality of life long before death.

Much like how diagnostic parameters for hypertension have been lowered, so have those for diabetes. A fasting glucose (twice or more) of above 126 mg/dL is now considered a diagnostic of diabetes. Since the fasting glucose is only a snapshot of a specific point in time, more physicians are looking to a test called the hemoglobin A1C, which measures the average glucose readings over a three-month period.

Number and Percentage of U.S. Population with Diagnosed Diabetes, 1958-2010

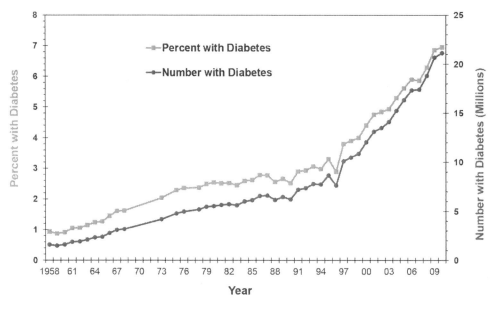

CDC's Division of Diabetes Translation. National Diabetes Surveillance System available at http://www.cdc.gov/diabetes/statistics

KNOW YOUR NUMBERS:

Normal:
A1C result of less than 5.7% *

Pre-diabetes:
A1C result between 5.7%–6.4%

Diabetes:
A1C of 6.5% and higher

*Personally, we like to see our patients with number that are 5.6% and lower.

Symptoms of diabetes can include excessive thirst, blurry vision, frequent urination, and fatigue. Because this disease comes on slowly, the symptoms often go unrecognized. The onset of diabetes is a slow process with the opportunity for us to turn back and correct health issues; but once the disease progresses to a certain point, the body begins to deteriorate quickly and permanent damage occurs. Getting a yearly exam, including diabetic screening, is critical to keeping the disease at bay.

DIABETIC COMPLICATIONS:

Heart disease
Stroke
High blood pressure
Blindness
Kidney disease
Neuropathy
Amputation

KNOW YOUR RISKS: Diabetes

___ Obesity or being overweight
___ High blood pressure
___ Family history
___ Sedentary lifestyle
___ Eating processed carbohydrates and sugary foods
___ Lack of fresh fruits and vegetables in the daily diet

___ High blood pressure
___ Polycystic ovary disease

SAVE YOURSELF:

___ Eat a nutritious diet
___ Exercise regularly
___ Keep your weight down, with waist size no greater than 40 inches for men and no greater than 35 inches for women
___ Avoid processed carbohydrates and refined sugars

DIAGNOSTIC MUST-HAVES:

___ Fasting glucose
___ Hemoglobin A1C
___ Autonomic Nervous System (ANS) testing if diabetic or pre-diabetic

Cancer

The second leading cause of death in the United States is cancer. Cancer cells start from regular healthy cells that have become defective or have mutated. From the day we are born our cells replicate; most replications are normal, but some are not. When our immune system is healthy and strong, any mutated cells are killed off, but when the mutations become too great or the immune system weakens, mutated cells become cancerous. Even healthy cells have a defined lifespan, and if they forget to die at the time they should or replicate too quickly, cancer can develop. Cancerous cells are also referred to as malignant cells. A diagnosis of cancer is always worrisome, but depending on the size, location, and type of cancer, the outlook may be very different. Since cancer can take many forms, for the sake of this chapter we will focus on the four leading cancers for both men and women in the United States: lung, colon, prostate (men), and breast cancers.

Lung cancer. Lung cancer is the deadliest form of cancer for men and women alike and claims more lives than breast, prostate, and colon cancers combined. Lung cancer comes in two major forms: small cell lung cancer (SCLC) and non–small cell lung cancer (NSCLC). It is possible for someone to have lung cancer that is made up of both types, but the most common form is NSCLC. At age 45, the risk for lung cancer becomes significant, but before that, it is rare. The leading cause of this type of cancer is smoking, and even people who have never smoked but are exposed to secondhand smoke increase their risk dramatically. The more a person smokes and the age they started smoking affects the risk ratio. It's important to understand that while the tobacco companies have used "low tar" as a marketing ploy, there is no evidence whatsoever that it reduces the risk of cancer.

"Down to their innate molecular core, cancer cells are hyperactive, survival-endowed, scrappy, fecund, inventive copies of ourselves."
—Siddhartha Mukherjee, *The Emperor of All Maladies*

The five-year survival rate for lung cancer when caught in the early stage and localized is 52.6%. Unfortunately, many lung cancer cases are not diagnosed until they reach an advanced stage; this is what makes screening so important. Once a patient is experiencing symptoms from lung cancer, the disease has often progressed. This is why over half the people with lung cancer will die within a year of being diagnosed. For every patient who has told us how they just can't quit smoking, there have been countless more that have shed a tear of regret once it's too late. Smokers can and should quit. Also, everyone should avoid secondhand smoke and refuse to let others' poor decision to smoke negatively affect their health. Whether you are a smoker or an innocent bystander, you do have a choice. Make the right one.

Colon cancer. One of the most regrettable diagnoses one can receive is colon cancer. That's because this type of cancer almost always starts as a noncancerous polyp. Polyps are small growths that can occur within the colon. Colon cancer screening can identify polyps long before they become malignant. Removing precancerous polyps can take the risk of colon cancer back down to zero. Colon cancer that does not originated from a polyp is rare. While colon cancer risk increases at 60 years of age, we have personally diagnosed many people, even as young as 34, with this deadly disease. It's important to understand that colon polyps do not cause symptoms, so they may exist without any warning whatsoever. If everyone was diligent about colon cancer screening, the rate of deaths from colon cancer could drop from being the second leading cause of cancer deaths straight down to the bottom of the list.

Colon cancer often starts in the innermost lining of the intestine, spreads throughout the colon, then to the lymph nodes and eventually to other organs. Catching this type of cancer in the earliest stages can mean a good prognosis; however, the ultimate goal is to remove any polyps prior to them ever turning cancerous in the first place. Late-stage colon cancer is often fatal. Prevention of colon cancer is easy, but it takes initiative. Although some people think colonoscopies are scary, they most likely have never witnessed the decline and death of a colon cancer patient. It's all about perspective. Dying of colon cancer is scary; having a colonoscopy is not.

Prostate cancer. The prostate is a walnut-sized gland that is part of the male reproductive system. It is partially a muscle and partially a gland. The purpose of the prostate is to secrete the slightly alkaline fluid that carries sperm. Because the gland has a dual purpose, its muscular action also helps push that fluid out through the urethra. When the prostate becomes enlarged, it can affect a man's ability to urinate properly. There are many different reasons that the prostate may become enlarged, and not all are cancerous.

Prostatitis, a condition in which the prostate gland becomes enlarged (usually due to infection), is fairly common and treatable with antibiotics. When men reach the age of 50, they often begin to see changes in their urine stream. This may be due to a condition known as benign prostatic hypertrophy (BPH). Just as the name suggests, BPH is not a form of cancer, nor does it pose an increased risk for cancer. However, if the symptoms become too bothersome, medications and surgical options are available.

Prostate cancer is rarely found in men under 40, but it is the most common cause of cancer deaths in men over 75. It occurs when cells within the prostate gland become cancerous. Treatment varies from surgery to radiation, hormone therapy, cryotherapy, and even chemotherapy. Sometimes, treatment will be delayed and doctors will opt for "watchful waiting." The controversy surrounding prostate cancer treatment is that some patients have this type of cancer and it never spreads, while others die despite treatment efforts. Because current science does not offer a way to differentiate between those patients who will beat the odds and those who won't, we recommend that every male be screened and understand their options.

Until recently, the only blood test available to screen for prostate cancer was the prostate-specific antigen (PSA) test. This test could not differentiate between BPH and the risk for prostate cancer, which was causing many men to go through unnecessary procedures in an effort to rule out cancer. The flip side of the problem: many physicians were less likely to move forward on a high PSA reading the first time because they have witnessed too many men go through unnecessary procedures. Now there is a more definitive test available: the PSA free and total. By adding the amount of free PSA, a calculation can be made using both numbers to arrive at a percentage likelihood of cancer. With only one in every 1,000 screenings requiring actual treatment, diagnosing is a tedious process, but one worthy of our energy and attention. We screen every patient, every year.

Breast cancer. While breast cancer is most common in women, it can affect men as well. When the tissues inside the breast start to change, a person will feel a swelling in a particular area or an identifiable lump. The two most common types of breast cancer among women are ductal carcinoma and lobular carcinoma. Ductal carcinoma is when the ducts that are designed to carry milk become cancerous. Lobular carcinoma is when the lobules, the part of the breast that makes milk, become cancerous. Ductal carcinoma is the more common of the two.

With the exception of non-melanoma skin cancer, breast cancer is the leading cause of cancer for women in the United States. Astoundingly, one in eight women will develop breast cancer in their lifetime. The BRCA1 and BRCA2 blood test that screen for specific types of breast cancer risk is available. (Note: this is a test to measure risk, not to diagnose cancer.) A positive test does not mean you will ever develop breast cancer from the mutation; likewise, a negative test does not mean there is not a risk of cancer. As much as 85% of breast cancer is found in women with no family history of the disease. However, if you have a first-degree relative with a history of breast cancer and you test positive, the risk ratio is exceptionally higher. Mammograms and self-examinations are still the number one tool for early detection.

KNOW YOUR RISKS: Cancer

___ Smoking or exposure to secondhand smoke

___ Exposure at home or work to certain chemicals or asbestos

___ Family history of cancer

___ Past radiation therapy

___ Personal history of precancerous conditions

___ History of inflammatory bowel disease (colon)

___ Dense breast tissue (breast)

___ Menstruation before age 12 (breast)

___ Diabetes

___ Chronic infection with hepatitis B or hepatitis C (liver)

___ Nonalcoholic fatty liver disease

___ Excessive alcohol consumption

___ Obesity

___ Diet low in vitamins and minerals

SAVE YOURSELF:

___ Eat seven serving of fresh fruits and vegetables per day

___ Do not smoke or expose yourself to secondhand smoke

___ Reduce stress levels

___ Exercise regularly

___ Maintain a low body fat percentage

___ Do not cook meats too long with extremely high heat

___ Limit the amount of meat intake, especially red meat

___ Eat a diet high in antioxidants

___ Avoid exposure to toxic chemicals

___ Avoid or limit alcohol

___ Avoid exposure to the sun. Use SPF 30 wide-spectrum sunscreen

___ Update your immunizations, including hepatitis immunizations

___ Practice safe sex

___ Do not ignore changes in your body or unusual symptoms
___ Have a yearly physical!

<u>DIAGNOSTIC MUST-HAVES:</u>

___ Stool for occult blood (usually done during your physical exam)
___ Colonoscopy or virtual colonography
___ PSA blood test, both free and total (for men)
___ Mammogram (for women)
___ CT of chest (smokers)

Infection

Over the years, medical advancements, especially the discovery and development of antibiotics and antiviral medications, have saved numerous lives. A person losing their life to infection was commonplace among all ages, whether it was from something contagious such as influenza, or bacterial complication from an injury. Many people watched their loved ones succumb to death long before they had a chance to live a full life.

Influenza and pneumonia. Influenza, often referred to as the flu, is a viral infection that attacks the respiratory tract. Symptoms may include fever, chills, runny or stuffy nose, aches, and sometimes intestinal upset. It has a long history, including the flu pandemic of 1918–1919. This particular strain, the Spanish flu, came on quickly. Many felt fine in the morning, but by nightfall they had passed away. During that year, an estimated 50 million people died worldwide, and about 675,000 of them were in the United States.

The vaccination for influenza, commonly referred to as the "flu shot," was created in the 1940s and was first used on soldiers in World War II. Around the 1960s, flu shots were being used in the general population, and the number of deaths each year dropped dramatically. Today, 36,000 people in the United States still die of the flu each year, mostly due to lack of vaccination. Influenza is not a simple form of infection and can lead to complications such as pneumonia. It's hard to believe that we still have deaths from influenza and pneumonia, but we do and together they make up the eighth leading cause of death in the United States.

Pneumonia is an inflammation of the lungs, often with infection. Pneumonia infection can be caused by bacteria, viruses, or fungus. It is often present in a patient who had a weakened immune system prior to exposure. Viral pneumonias tend to heal on their own, but bacterial and fungal lung infections can be serious and life threatening. Shockingly, there are over 90 types of pneumococcal bacteria. The pneumonia vaccine was first produced in 1977 and has changed over the years, but it still doesn't cover all strains of pneumonia. However, vaccinations against pneumonia save countless lives each year. In most recent years, the vaccine was effective for six years; however, in 2012 it was released as a one-shot lifelong vaccination.

KNOW YOUR RISKS:

____ Exposure to those with the flu
____ Age—young children and those over 65 are more likely to contract the flu
____ Compromised immune system
____ Live in a dorm, apartment, assisted living center, or nursing home
____ Healthcare worker
____ Visit or stay in a hospital during flu season
____ Have a chronic illness such as diabetes, heart disease, asthma, or COPD
____ Pregnant

SAVE YOURSELF:

____ Get a flu shot
____ Avoid crowds
____ Use hand sanitizer and wash hands frequently
____ Use sanitizing wipes on door handles, grocery store carts, and other shared items
____ Never share food or drink with others
____ Get at least 7.5 hours of sleep a night
____ Exercise regularly (avoid public gyms during the flu season)
____ Eat at least seven servings of fresh fruits/fresh vegetables per day
____ Get a flu shot yearly and a one-time pneumonia vaccine
____ Get vaccinated for hepatitis A and B

DIAGNOSTIC MUST-HAVES:

___ If symptomatic, test for influenza A and B
___ Chest X-ray if pneumonia is suspected
___ A blood count may also be ordered by your healthcare provider

---

Super-Charge Your Immune System

A healthy smoothie will help you start your morning right. We always recommend a blend of fruits and vegetables to power-boost your immune system. This is our favorite combination (makes 2 glasses):

2 ½ cups of mango nectar
2 large leafs of organic kale
5 red raspberries
3 strawberries
1 cup of fresh or frozen blueberries

Blend for 1–2 minutes. Any left over will keep in the fridge for 24 hours.

HIV and AIDS. Human immunodeficiency virus (HIV) was first recognized in 1981. Since that time, there has been much confusion between HIV and acquired immune deficiency syndrome (AIDS). HIV is the initial virus and AIDS is the complications that result from being infected with HIV. There are two types of HIV in the United States: HIV-1 and HIV-2. HIV-1 is the most common and will be referred to throughout this section.

HIV attacks the immune system, specifically destroying CD4$^+$ T cells which are critical in protecting the body against infection. When the CD4$^+$ T cells reach a particularly low level, the patient is considered to have AIDS. Early HIV infection should be treated because if left untreated, it can lead to other complications, including cardiovascular disease, kidney disease, liver disease, and cancer. Sometimes, there are no initial symptoms of HIV, and other times, those infected will just feel like they have flu for a while and then the symptoms will go away.

Every 9.5 minutes, someone in the United States is infected with HIV, and one in five people who have HIV are unaware they have been infected. HIV is not just an infection that affects the homosexual male population; it affects both male and female, both homosexual and heterosexual, and people of all ages. It has been reported in all 50 U.S. states. Unfortunately, people have become complacent about HIV infection, especially our youth who are often participating in promiscuous sexual activity. The U.S. CDC estimates that more than half of all undiagnosed HIV infections are the youth aged 13–24. As a parent, this should be a wakeup call. We must educate our younger folks of the dangers that come from sexual activity and drug use.

Just as our youth needs to be educated, so do people of all ages, even those in their second half of life. Seniors are also at an increased risk because they are less likely to use protection. Because of advancements in medicine, many people who originally contracted HIV in their younger years have been able to live seemingly healthy lives. The medications can control the virus, but there is no cure for HIV. A person on antiviral medications for HIV can still infect others. Promiscuity and drug use is a source of possible infection for all, regardless of age, race, or socioeconomic class. The CDC recommends that healthcare providers routinely screen for HIV in those aged 13–64, and repeat the screening at least annually for those at high risk.

KNOW YOUR RISKS:

____ Injecting drugs or steroids through shared needles

____ Unprotected vaginal, anal, or oral sex

____ Men having sex with men; multiple or anonymous partners

____ Exchanging sex for drugs or money

____ Diagnosed with or treated for hepatitis, tuberculosis, or a sexually transmitted disease, such as syphilis

____ Unprotected sex with someone whose history is unknown

SAVE YOURSELF:

____ Stay monogamous and avoid having sex (oral, anal, and vaginal) except with a single non-infected partner (sex only within a committed relationship)

___ Never use a shared or non-sterile needle

___ Protect yourself at all times from the body fluids of others (healthcare workers should take extra precautions)

DIAGNOSTIC MUST-HAVES:

___ HIV blood test

Hepatitis. Hepatitis, or inflammation of the liver, can occur for many reasons, but most often it is caused by a virus. The viral infection has three prevalent forms: hepatitis A (HAV), hepatitis B (HBV), and hepatitis C (HCV). The most commonly occurring strain in the United States, HCV, is also the most serious, killing thousands of people every year.

Currently, it's estimated that 4.1 million Americans are infected with HCV. Transmission can occur through the sharing of drug needles or having unprotected sex. An infected mother can also pass the disease along to her baby. Although there is no cure or vaccine for HCV, there is a medication treatment that is effective for some people.

A person with hepatitis may not exhibit symptoms, which is why so many people remain unaware that they have the disease. However, they can still transmit the virus to others even if they are symptom-free. Symptoms, when present, can include jaundice, fever, nausea, and abdominal pain.

KNOW YOUR RISKS:

___ Unprotected vaginal, anal, or oral sex with multiple partners, anonymous partners, or anyone who is at risk

___ Sharing razors or toothbrushes

___ Using intravenous drugs

___ Getting a tattoo or body piercing

___ Unwashed hands after using the restroom

SAVE YOURSELF:

___ Stay monogamous and avoid having sex (oral, anal, and vaginal) except with a single non-infected partner (sex only within a committed relationship)

___ Avoid recreational drugs, especially intravenous ones

____ Avoid tattoos

____ Wash hand after using the restroom

____ Never share anything that could come in contact with body fluids

____ Healthcare workers and some other professions should take extra precautions to avoid contact with body fluids

DIAGNOSTIC MUST-HAVES:

____ Hepatitis laboratory testing

Stress. Stress is never listed as the cause of death on a death certificate, nor does it appear on the mortality charts and graphs of the CDC; however, its effects on the death rate may be the most potent and far reaching of all of the killers listed above. A condition rather than a disease, its modus operandi is to weaken the immune system over time, leaving the body more susceptible to illness. When the body is in stress mode, it shifts its primary focus from growth and repair to survival. Everything from the digestive tract to the skin is compromised. Our bodies are designed to use the fight-or-flight reaction as an instinct of survival when danger is present. We were not created to handle large amounts of constant stress. Unfortunately, lifestyles today often come with continuous stress, leaving the body in an ongoing state of fight or flight.

When the body feels stress, it undergoes physiological changes, disturbing the nervous, immune, musculoskeletal, and endocrine systems. Stress causes the blood vessels to constrict, blood pressure and pulse to rise, and the body to be flooded with hormones, such as cortisol and adrenaline. Over time, this overtaxes the body and causes premature aging to take place. Indirectly, stress causes a number of diseases. For example, high cortisol levels cause weight gain, especially around the middle; this additional weight increases the risk of diabetes. Weight gain and heart disease can also come from sleep deprivation, a known side effect of stress.

New technology has allowed us to see how stress can affect the aging process on a cellular level. We know that substantial or constant stress leads to shortening of the telomeres. Telomeres, the ends of the DNA strands on our chromosomes, are necessary for life. The strands must remain long enough for continued cell replication so that new cells can replace old cells. Once these telomeres shorten, so does your life. (See telomere diagram on page 70.)

Stress presents outward signs of the inward damage. Symptoms of stress include depression, anxiety, weight gain, skin irritations, headaches, change in appetite, change in mood, frequent illness, and aches or pains. These symptoms should not be brushed off; consider them a caution flag that something needs to change.

Sometimes stress can't be avoided, so finding ways to manage it is critical. Stressors will have less of an effect if the body is getting proper nutrition and regular exercise. These things help stave off the ill effects of the hormone influx and also help improve immunity. Journaling is an effective stress buster, and studies show it helps reduce anxiety and improve sleep. Take charge of your health by cultivating stress management techniques that work for you.

KNOW YOUR RISKS:

____ High-pressure job
____ Financial pressures
____ Relationship difficulties
____ Doing too much
____ Divorce
____ Death of a loved one
____ Perfectionism
____ Chronic procrastination

SAVE YOURSELF:

____ Exercise daily
____ Eat a balanced diet
____ Avoid caffeine
____ Never consume "energy" drinks
____ Avoid artificial sweeteners
____ Journal
____ Do yoga

___ Manage expectations

___ Create and stick to a budget

___ Mend fences and be slow to criticize others

___ Do not over-schedule

___ Find a job you enjoy or learn to enjoy the one you have

DIAGNOSTIC MUST-HAVES:

___ Blood pressure check

___ Complete physical exam yearly

___ Autonomic nervous system (ANS) test

___ Telomere testing

___ Micronutrient testing

STRESS EFFECTS ON THE BODY

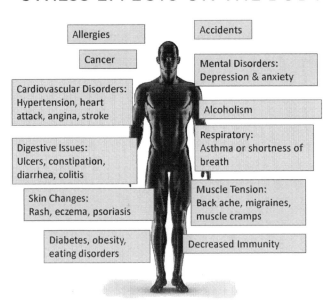

CHAPTER SIX

THE AVAT FACTOR

Knowing your real age

"The doctor of the future will give no medication, but will interest his patients in the care of the human frame, diet, and in the cause and prevention of disease." —Thomas A. Edison

---

In 1952, Dr. Virginia Apgar, the founder of neonatology, conducted an evaluation designed to measure the effects that anesthesia had on babies during childbirth. She used five different factors: skin color, pulse rate, reflex, muscle tone, and breathing. The Apgar score is still widely used today as a way to score the health of a newborn baby—the first time that our overall health is assessed and scored. Doctors measure many things on an individual scale, looking at various things such as blood work, EKGs, and so forth, but they never really assess the patient using an all-encompassing score.

ANS, VO2Max, Advanced Lipid Panel, and Telomeres

We have found that a number of tests are critical in determining a patient's health and likelihood of aging well. That's why we have developed a method that measures different systems within the body and gives an overall scaled score. Named after the different tests that are used in the formula (ANS, VO2Max, Advanced Lipid Panel, and Telomeres), we call it the AVAT Factor. The purpose of the AVAT is to determine whether a patient is on target with their age or in better or worse health than expected. The results are a great motivator for doctors and patients alike, because it helps determine the areas of strength and weakness. People often say they want to live a long time, but don't really know where to start. Knowing the areas that require work and taking steps to improve in those areas will increase the chances for a long and healthy life.

The Tests

Autonomic nervous system (ANS) testing. When most people think of stress, they think of busy schedules, deadlines, and pressures. Stress actually comes in three forms: physical, mental, or a combination of the two. When a person is exposed to long-term negative factors, whether it be physical overload, or harmful lifestyle behaviors such as tobacco, alcohol, or improper nutrition, the body is put into a state of physical stress. Family problems, feelings of insecurity or inadequacy, and even idleness can cause mental stress. In a worst-case scenario, mental and physical stresses occur simultaneously for a prolonged amount of time. When this happens, the body has no choice but to fight back.

The body elicits a response through the autonomic nervous system (ANS). This system is divided up into two parts: the sympathetic nervous system and the parasympathetic nervous system. Of equal importance, these systems work to keep each other, and the body as a whole, in balance. The sympathetic nervous system is in action during times of danger or excitement when adrenaline jolts through the body, like an electrical shock. The parasympathetic nervous system, on the other hand, is less noticeable, and works continuously in the background to ensure that the body functions properly. The systems should be equally balanced, without one having to work harder than the other. Measuring this balance can help determine overall health as well as determine how a person's autonomic nervous system is aging.

Because chronological age is not a determination of overall health, tests like this help healthcare providers determine a functional age. The functional age, as determined by the ANS testing, takes into account the physiological, mental, and emotional strain that is placed on the autonomic nervous system. When the parasympathetic and sympathetic systems are out of equilibrium, a person will have a functional age that is higher than their chronological age. Premature aging puts a person at risk for developing life-threatening diseases, like those mentioned in Chapter 5.

VO2Max stress test. True physical fitness can be determined by measuring a person's maximum oxygen consumption, what is commonly termed VO2Max. This test indexes the level of physical fitness by measuring the maximum amount of oxygen the body can use while exercising. Muscles need oxygen to function properly, and it takes a number of body parts, including the heart, lungs, blood vessels, and muscles, to transform and transport oxygen (supplied by the air we breathe) to the muscles and other body parts. Our muscles require oxygen to do physical work—the more oxygen, the longer they can perform without fatigue. When a person exercises regularly, the body becomes more efficient at transporting and utilizing oxygen. On the flip side, a sedentary lifestyle will prevent the body from functioning at a higher capacity.

Exercise stress testing with VO2Max looks at the functional capacity of the heart and lungs and how well they work together. A good test will measure and report a number of items, including:

- Maximum oxygen consumption
- Maximum heart rate
- Resting and maximum blood pressure
- Cardiovascular risks such as a Framingham Pre-test Vascular Age
- Comparative aerobic fitness for chronological age
- Class rank of VO2Max functional capacity, with Class 1 being optimal
- Basal metabolic rate (BMR), the number of daily calories required to maintain current weight
- Metabolic equivalent of tasks (METS), the rate at which true exercise is achieved
- The number of pounds that can be lifted before there is a change in heart rate or blood pressure

From the results of the above tests, a healthcare provider can determine a patient's cardiopulmonary health and fitness level. The report should define the Post-test Cardiovascular Risk, the heart age versus chronological age, and the aerobic fitness percentile. A person who is aging on target or better than normal will have a low risk for cardiovascular disease, a Framingham Pre-test Vascular Age that is close to their chronological age, and fall into the Class 1 VO2Max Functional Capacity.

Advanced lipid panel. For years, healthcare providers have relied on four basic lipid panel numbers: total cholesterol, LDL (bad cholesterol), HDL (good cholesterol), and triglycerides. Some patients with normal or slightly high cholesterol numbers have heart attacks, while others with extremely high numbers appear healthy without experiencing any serious cardiac events. This paradox used to leave medical professionals baffled. The mystery was solved with the discovery that LDL cholesterol particles come in different shapes and sizes.

An advanced lipid panel gives information about all the particles of cholesterol and triglycerides, providing a clearer picture of the risk of future disease or cardiovascular events. There are a number of different advanced lipid panel options that physicians use. We prefer the Berkley test, which was designed by Berkley HeartLab, but other tests include the VAP and NMR LipoProfile. Each of these tests will give the most significant piece of information: the LDL particle size.

LDL particle size may be categorized as Pattern A, which is large and buoyant, or Pattern B, which is small and dense. The small and dense particles are the most dangerous—they can penetrate the lining of the arteries and aggregate, and this is what causes a decrease in blood flow. Most people are under the impression that the buildup, also referred to as plaque, reaches 100% blockage, causing a heart attack. While the plaque leads to the problem, a heart attack is actually caused when a part of the plaque breaks off, or ruptures, and a blood clot forms, acting like a cork in the artery. This explains how a person can be walking around fine one moment and the next minute find themselves in the emergency room—or worse yet, the morgue.

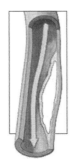
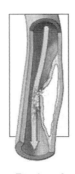
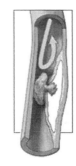

Plaque   Ruptured   Blood Clot Forms,
                Plaque   Blocking Flow

Smoking, poor diet, and lack of exercise can all increase the likelihood for having Pattern B LDL cholesterol. This pattern causes a threefold greater risk for coronary heart disease or a cardiovascular event. The good news is that Pattern B can be converted to Pattern A through lifestyle changes. This is exactly why people need to have advanced lipid panels performed to understand their risks. Again, you can't fix what you don't measure.

Telomere testing. In 2009, the Nobel Prize in Physiology or Medicine was given to Carol Greider of John Hopkins School of Medicine, Elizabeth Blackburn of the University of California–Berkeley, and Harvard geneticist Jack Szostak for their pioneering research on telomeres and chromosomes and for the discovery Greider and Blackburn made 15 years prior when they found telomerase. The work of these brilliant minds changed the way physicians and scientist would forever look at aging and disease.

Every single cell in the body contains a nucleus. Within the nucleus are 46 strands of chromosomes. These strands are paired up to include DNA from both the mother and the father. Each time the cell replicates, it loses a bit of its length. Because a cell requires all pairs to be present during replication, the ends of the chromosomes contain long pairs of the DNA sequence TTAGGG, which have the sole purpose of protecting the functional DNA. These protective pairs can deteriorate without harming the integrity of the cell, but once they are used up, the cell is at risk for mutation or death.

An embryo has approximately 15,000 base pairs in each telomere, but by the time it has been delivered as a newborn, that number has decreased to approximately 10,000 base pairs. Therefore, the aging process begins long before we are placed in our mother's arms.

Telomeres on chromosomes are like a wicks on a candle. Just like candles burn at different rates, so do our telomeres, and once they are expended, the cells die. Likewise, in the book *The Immortal Edge*, Fossel, Blackburn, and Woynarowski refer to telomeres as the plastic wraps at the end of shoe laces. They protect the laces, but once they are worn down, the laces fray and begin to fall apart.

Two people with the same chronological age will have different telomere lengths depending on their overall body health. A number of studies have shown that shorter telomeres are a sign of advanced aging. Things like inflammation, smoking, poor diet, and lack of exercise all shorten telomeres and lead to cell death. Not all telomeres in the body shorten at the same rate; some groups may shorten at a quicker rate than others.

When the telomeres of cells come to the end, the cells go into a state of retirement or death wherein they can no longer reproduce. This stage is referred to as senescence. Many people have experienced this deterioration in a part of their body, such as cartilage in a joint. These cells have reached that stage of retirement. The bigger problem with senescence is that these cells can negatively affect good tissues around them by secreting harmful proteins. While this is the cause of advanced aging, it can also be a precursor to cancer.

For anyone wishing to prevent aging, the main goal should be to monitor and promote healthy telomere length. Telomere length is the age of the body at the smallest level: the cellular level. It's like looking at one's age through a microscope, much more scientific than a chronological number.

We measure telomeres using the SpectraCell® telomere test. Telomere scores are calculated based on average telomere length in peripheral whole blood cells. This average is then compared to telomere lengths from a population sample in the same age range, giving the patient's percentile score, or age, at the cellular level.

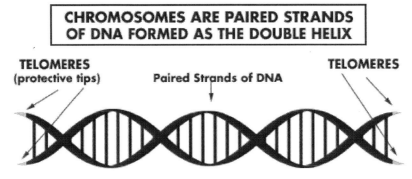

CHROMOSOMES ARE PAIRED STRANDS OF DNA FORMED AS THE DOUBLE HELIX

TELOMERES (protective tips)   Paired Strands of DNA   TELOMERES

How the Scoring Works

Chronological age is used as a starting point for the scoring. If results show a person to be older than their chronological age, they will have a negative subfactor, and if they are younger than their chronological age, they will have a positive subfactor. A functional age that matches the chronological age receives a score of 0. Unlike tests that give an age-related result, an advanced lipid panel shows either a Pattern A, Pattern B, or Pattern AB, describing the particle size of LDL cholesterol. Pattern A receives a +1, and Pattern B is a –1. If the patient has pattern AB, meaning some of each, they still receive a –1. The chart below details the scoring system. Subfactors are added together to create a total AVAT Factor Score.

AVAT SCORING

Functional Age > Chronological Age			Test	Functional Age < Chronological Age		
Over 15	Over 10	Over 5		Under 5	Under 10	Under 15
-3	-2	-1	ANS	1	2	3
-3	-2	-1	VO2Max	1	2	3
		-1	Adv. lipid	1		
-3	-2	-1	Telomere	1	2	3

As you can see from the AVAT Scoring chart, the best possible score is a perfect 10 and the lowest possible score is a –10. It's unlikely that many people will reach a perfect score, but the goal is to have an AVAT score that is positive, or at the very least 0, which would be in line with the chronological age. Results falling on the negative side of the chart indicate that the body has begun to age prematurely in that area.

Feeling a little overwhelmed? It's always easier to understand a concept when using examples. The following cases represent common findings in patients. As you can see, lifestyle plays a large role in the aging process.

AVAT Example #1

John is a 61-year-old man who has a strong family history of heart disease, and has taken above-average care of himself through diet and a healthy lifestyle. He does not drink or smoke. He works long hours and does not exercise as much as he should, averaging only one to two times per week. He has not suffered any major illnesses. His ANS shows his functional age to be 59. According to his VO2Max, his vascular age is 61 and he is in Functional Class 1. The advanced lipid panel shows his choles-terol to be 220, but it is all Pattern A. His telomere test gives him a cellular age of 55.

AVAT SCORING

Functional Age > Chronological Age			Test	Functional Age < Chronological Age		
Over 15	Over 10	Over 5		Under 5	Under 10	Under 15
			ANS	1		
			VO2Max	1		
			Adv. lipid	1		
			Telomere		2	

With a total AVAT Factor score of +5, John is aging slower than expected. This is more than likely due to his lifestyle choices. That being said, he has room to improve and can likely raise his AVAT score even higher through increasing his exercise routine to three to four times a week. More than likely, this will improve both his ANS and his VO2Max results. (Note: current VO2Max is 0 because it matches his chronological age.)

AVAT Example #2

Mary is 46 years old. She has a strong family history of diabetes and has had high blood sugar levels in the past, but has always remained right on the edge of having pre-diabetes. She has a job that keeps her at a desk for seven to eight hours a day. She drinks on occasion, but nothing regular. Her tobacco history includes a pack-a-day habit that ended about five years ago. She tries to get to the gym at least three days a week now, but this is a relatively new endeavor. Her ANS showed some stiffening of the arteries and a functional age of 54. VO2Max results showed her to be in Func-tional Class 2 with a vascular age of 55, and in poorer shape than others her age. Her advanced lipid panel showed her cholesterol to be 210, but she was Pattern AB. Her telomere testing showed that her cellular age was 60.

AVAT SCORING

Functional Age > Chronological Age			Test	Functional Age < Chronological Age		
Over 15	Over 10	Over 5		Under 5	Under 10	Under 15
		-1	ANS			
		-1	VO2Max			
		-1	Adv. lipid			
	-2		Telomere			

Her total AVAT Factor score is –6, showing that her lifestyle choices and sedentary job have caused her body to deteriorate faster than others with the same chronological age. While her telomere score is not anticipated to move too far toward the positive side, she may be able to slow further shortening of her telomeres by using resveratrol and astragalus root supplements, as described later in this chapter. With continued regular exercise, VO2Max results should improve. Depending on the damage caused by her previous smoking, ANS results may or may not improve. Through regular exercise, she can convert her AB Pattern to all A. Mary will never reach the perfect +10, but it's not too late to slow the aging process significantly. She can still possibly reach a score of 0 or even a low positive number.

The purpose of the AVAT Factor score is to give patients and their healthcare providers an easy way to assess their level of aging, and offer targeted, specific ways to improve health. By looking at the effects of aging in a detailed manner and approaching improvements in a measurable and scientific way, healthcare providers can objectively track their patients' progress.

Making Improvements

It's pointless to measure something unless you intend to offer a means for improvement. Just as patients want a treatment, not only a diagnosis, the AVAT Factor score is a tool for improvement, not a final verdict. The score is not final until the patient is doing everything possible to achieve the highest achievable result given their individual potential. For some people, success comes at a score of 0, while others achieve it at 8 or 9. A lucky few will reach a perfect 10.

ANS improvement. The best way to improve the autonomic nervous system is to use it often and protect it through exercise, hydration, and good nutrition. Exercising at least three times a week and doing cardiovascular, muscle-building, and flexibility exercises will help greatly toward this end. Proper hydration, for example, is critical to improved autonomic function. By taking the body weight number in pounds and dividing that number in half, the required number of ounces of water per day can be determined. Drink a minimum of this amount per day, and even more if exercising or in dry or hot climates. Nutrition can be improved by incorporating seven servings of fresh fruits/vegetables per day into your diet. Micronutrient deficiencies are commonly found in those with a low ANS functional age; therefore, taking pharmaceutical-grade supplements can prevent such deficiencies and optimize important nutrient levels.

VO2Max improvement. Each VO2Max will include the number of METs that a patient can exercise effectively at. Reaching that peak at least three times per week for at least 30 minutes will help improve the vascular fitness level and improve VO2Max scores, helping the body utilize oxygen more effectively. Smoking any sort of tobacco should be stopped and alcohol consumption limited if not completely omitted.

Advanced lipid panel improvements. Nutrition is an important part of a healthy lipid profile. Eat lean meat, lots of leafy green vegetables, and avoid fat and processed carbohydrates. Even with a perfect diet, the LDL pattern is actually most affected by exercise. Regular exercise is the best way to keep LDL particle size within the desired Pattern A size. By avoiding Pattern B, the body will decrease the chances of a possibly life-threatening vascular event.

Telomere improvements. Regular exercise, good nutrition, and good lifestyle choices all help keep telomeres from shortening too quickly. Taking supplements such as resveratrol and astragalus root have been shown to protect telomeres. In some schools of thought, these supplements also help increase telomerase and therefore lengthen telomeres as well, and prevent them from shortening.

Su[180] pplementology

Supplements can be confusing, especially with all the advertising targeted at the middle-aged demographic. The fear of looking or feeling "old" drives the worldwide multibillion-dollar anti-aging market. In order to simplify things, we have constructed a list of the supplements that we feel are essential to good health as we age. These are the same supplements that we take ourselves and that we recommend to our patients.

Remember that all supplements should be pharmaceutical grade; this is the only way to ensure that the ingredients actually match what the label states. The FDA does not regulate supplements the same way that they regulate food and drugs. Manufacturers do not need to register their products with FDA or get FDA approval before producing or selling dietary supplements.

Amino acids	Higher total strength and lean body mass scores. Elevated biologically active growth hormone. We recommend: N-acetyl-L-cysteine (750 mg) L-glutamine (500 mg) L-ornithine HCl (450) L-arginine HCl (600 mg) L-lysine HCl (600 mg)
Astragalus root	Used in Chinese medicine for centuries, astragalus has antibacterial and anti-inflammatory properties. Builds up the immune system and helps fight off diseases associated with premature aging. We recommend: astragalus herbal extract (500 mg) with astragalus (50 mg)
CoQ10	Necessary for cell growth and maintenance. Functions as an antioxidant. We recommend: natural coenzyme Q10 (30 mg)

Omega 3	Essential fatty acids that boost heart health and lower triglycerides. Some people find relief from arthritis and depression as well. We recommend: EPA (660 mg) and DHA (340 mg)
Multivitamin	Not all multivitamins are the same. Some are better for aging than others. We recommend: pharmaceutical-grade supplement that includes a minimum of vitamins A, Bs, C, E, as well as folic acid, pantothenic acid, copper, magnesium, chromium, potassium, and ginkgo biloba
Resveratrol	Promotes cell energy. Also triggers proteins that rejuvenate cells. Hold great promise in anti-aging. We recommend: 200 mg as trans-resveratrol
Vitamin D	Important to overall body function. Studies have proven that a low Vitamin D level is associated with increased mortality. We recommend: 5000 IU

The Stay Young Vitamin line is a great way to ensure you are getting what you need. Supplements from this pharmaceutical-grade line can be purchased by going to www.stayyoungvitamins.com or by calling (800) 910-3932.

CHAPTER SEVEN

THE FUEL OF LIFE

Micronutrients and a healthy body

"Let food be thy medicine, thy medicine shall be thy food." —Hippocrates

The complexity of the human body is such a mystery that it may never be fully understood. Good health and longevity begins at the cellular level, and cells need proper fuel through a delicate balance of nutrients. Our food is our fuel, but like the gasoline we put in our cars, not all food is created equally. Sometimes, when certain nutrients fall below optimal levels, symptoms appear, and when those levels drop too low, the body is unable to function properly and starts to break down. Vitamin, mineral, and antioxidant deficiencies can lead to inflammatory processes and malfunctions of the immune system. Among other things, this can lead to cardiovascular disease, arthritis, diabetes, and cancer.

Many factors can affect micronutrient levels. Even well-intended individuals who eat right, exercise, and take supplements can still become deficient. Each person's biochemical makeup and metabolism determines their specific requirements. Because needs change as bodies age, more or less of certain nutrients at different stages of life are required. Changes in lifestyle may also dictate the required amounts of different vitamins, minerals, or antioxidants. All of these factors work in conjunction to create a personal micronutrient profile as unique as a fingerprint.

Western medicine has only just started to grasp the concept that cultures have taken into account for many generations: micronutrient deficiencies are at the root of most symptoms and diseases. Many healthcare providers look to these deficiencies as an afterthought rather than a starting point, often leaving patients with unnecessary prescriptions and high medical bills. Worse yet, many don't even look for these deficiencies at all; therefore, the patient may never have a proper diagnosis.

Headaches, weight gain, pain, insomnia, impotence, fibromyalgia, fatigue, and even asthma are commonly treated by identifying and correcting micronutrient deficiencies. Why, then, have most people never heard of micronutrient testing? A partial answer is that many physicians don't realize they can test for all of these levels, or they feel the tests would be cost prohibitive. The more likely reason is that many healthcare providers are unaware that these nutrients can now be tested within the cell, and not just in the serum.

In the past, serum blood tests would give a general idea of the nutrient levels, but could not tell the healthcare provider if the body was able to utilize a particular nutrient effectively. For example, a low nutrient level may still fall within the normal range in the serum test, but the patient could have symptoms. Also, serum test results could change significantly based on recent dietary intake. Now, with the use of technology offered through SpectraCell Laboratories, Inc., micronutrients can be measured on a cellular level, providing a more accurate snapshot. The real challenge that lies ahead is educating healthcare providers about micronutrients, their importance, and how to properly correct deficiencies.

Micronutrient Chart

Nutrient/Function	Where It Is Found	Deficiency Symptoms/ Problems
Vitamin E: Antioxidant; regulates oxidation reactions; stabilizes cell membrane; immune function; protects against cardiovascular disease, cataracts, and macular degeneration	Wheat germ, liver, eggs, nuts, seeds, cold-pressed vegetable oils, dark leafy greens, sweet potatoes, avocados, asparagus	Unhealthy skin or hair, rupturing or red blood cells, anemia, bruising, PMS, hot flashes, eczema, psoriasis, cataracts, compromised wound healing, muscle weakness, sterility

The Fuel of Life

Nutrient/Function	Where It Is Found	Deficiency Symptoms/ Problems
Calcium: Strengthens bones and teeth; helps heart, nerves, muscles, body systems work properly; needs other nutrients to function	Dairy, wheat/soy flour, molasses, brewer's yeast, Brazil nuts, broccoli, cabbage, dark leafy greens, hazelnuts, oysters, sardines, canned salmon	Osteoporosis, osteomalacia, osteoarthritis, muscle cramps, irritability, acute anxiety, colon cancer risk
Chromium: Assists insulin function; increases fertility; carbohydrate/fat metabolism; essential for fetal growth/development	Brewer's yeast, whole grains, seafood, green beans, broccoli, prunes, nuts, potatoes, meat	Metabolic syndrome, insulin resistance, decreased fertility
Magnesium: Responsible for over 300 biochemical reactions; muscle/ nerve function; heart rhythm; immune system; strong bones; regulates calcium, copper, zinc, potassium, and vitamin D	Green vegetables, beans, peas, nuts, seeds, whole unprocessed grains	Loss of appetite, nausea, vomiting, fatigue, cramps, numbness, tingling, seizures, heart spasms, personality changes, irregular heart rhythm
Selenium: Antioxidant; works with Vitamin E; immune function; prostaglandin production	Brewer's yeast, wheat germ, liver, butter, cold-water fish, shellfish, garlic, whole grains, sunflower seeds, Brazil nuts	Destruction of heart and pancreas, sore muscles, fragility of red blood cells, compromised immune system
Zinc: Supports enzymes; immune system; wound healing; taste/ smell; DNA synthesis; normal growth and development during pregnancy, childhood, and adolescence	Oysters, red meat, poultry, beans, nuts, seafood, whole grains, fortified breakfast cereals, dairy	Growth retardation, hair loss, diarrhea, impotence, eye and skin lesions, loss of appetite, loss of taste, weight loss, compromised wound healing, mental lethargy

Nutrient/Function	Where It Is Found	Deficiency Symptoms/ Problems
CoQ10: Powerful antioxidant; stops oxidation of LDL cholesterol; energy production; important to heart, liver, and kidneys	Oily fish, organ meats, whole grains	Congestive heart failure, high blood pressure, angina, mitral valve prolapse, fatigue, gingivitis, compromised immune system, stroke, cardiac arrhythmias
Carnitine: Energy; heart function; oxidizes amino acids for energy; metabolizes ketones	Red meat, dairy, fish, poultry, tempeh (fermented soybeans), wheat, asparagus, avocados, peanut butter	Elevated cholesterol, suboptimal liver function, muscle weakness, reduced energy, impaired glucose control
N-Acetyl-L-cysteine (NAC) and Glutathione: Glutathione production; lowers homocysteine and lipoprotein (a); heals lungs; reduces inflammation; decreases muscle fatigue; liver detoxification; immune function	Meats, ricotta, cottage cheese, yogurt, wheat germ, granola, oat flakes	Free-radical overload, elevated homocysteine, increased cancer risk, cataracts, macular degeneration, compromised immune function, prohibits toxin elimination
Alpha lipoic acid: Energy,; blood flow to nerves; glutathione levels in brain; insulin sensitivity; effectiveness of vitamins C, E, and antioxidants	Supplementation, spinach, broccoli, beef, brewer's yeast, some organ meats	Diabetic neuropathy, reduced muscle mass, atherosclerosis, Alzheimer's, failure to thrive, brain atrophy, high lactic acid
Copper: Bone formation; involved in healing process; energy production; hair and skin coloring; taste sensitivity; stimulates iron absorption; helps metabolize several fatty acids	Oysters, seeds, dark leafy vegetables, organ meats, dried legumes, whole grains, breads, nuts, shellfish, chocolate, soybeans, oats, blackstrap molasses	Osteoporosis, anemia, baldness, diarrhea, general weakness, impaired respiratory function, myelopathy, decreased skin pigment, reduced resistance to infection

Nutrient/Function	Where It Is Found	Deficiency Symptoms/ Problems
Vitamin B1: Carbohydrate conversion; breaks down fats and protein; digestion; nervous system; skin; hair; eyes; mouth; liver; immune system	Pork, organ meats, whole-grain and enriched cereals, brown rice, wheat germ, bran brewer's yeast, blackstrap molasses	Heart disease, age-related cognitive decline, Alzheimer's, fatigue
Vitamin B2: Metabolism; carbohydrate conversion; breaks down fats and protein; digestion; nervous system; skin; hair; eyes; mouth; liver	Brewer's yeast, almonds, organ meats, whole grains, wheat germ, mushrooms, soy, dairy, eggs, green vegetables	Anemia, decreased free radical protection, cataracts, poor thyroid function, B6 deficiency, fatigue, elevated homocysteine
Vitamin B3: Energy; digestion; nervous system; skin; hair; eyes; liver; eliminates toxins; sex/stress	Beets, brewer's yeast, meat, poultry, organ meats, fish, seeds, nuts	Cracking and scaling skin, digestive problems, confusion, anxiety, fatigue
Vitamin B6: Hormone regulation; improves circulation; enzymes; protein metabolism; red blood cell production; reduces homocysteine; nerve and muscle cells, DNA/RNA; B12 absorption; immune function	Poultry, tuna, salmon, shrimp, beef liver, lentils, soybeans, seeds, nuts, avocados, bananas, carrots, brown rice, bran, wheat, germ, whole-grain flour	Depression, sleep and skin problems, confusion, anxiety, fatigue
Vitamin B12: Healthy nerve cells; DNA/ RNA; red blood cell production; iron function	Fish, meat, poultry, eggs, milk, milk products	Anemia, fatigue, constipation, loss of appetite/weight, numbness and tingling in the hands and feet, depression, dementia, poor memory, oral soreness
Biotin: Carbohydrates; fat; amino acid metabolism (the building blocks of protein)	Salmon, meats, vegetables, grains, legumes, lentils, egg yolks, milk, sweet potatoes, seeds, nuts, wheat germ	Depression, compromised nervous system, premature graying, hair, skin

Nutrient/Function	Where It Is Found	Deficiency Symptoms/ Problems
Folate: Mental health; infant DNA/ RNA; adolescence and pregnancy; with B12, regulates red blood cell production and iron function. Reduces homocysteine levels	Supplementation, fortified grains, tomato juice, green vegetables, black-eyed peas, lentils, beans	Anemia, immune function, fatigue, insomnia, unhealthy or loss of hair, high homocysteine, cardiovascular disease
Pantothenate: Red blood cell production; sex and stress-related hormone regulation; immune function; healthy digestion; helps body use other vitamins	Meat, vegetables, whole grains, legumes, lentils, egg yolks, milk, sweet potatoes, seeds, nuts, wheat germ, salmon	Stress tolerance, wound healing, skin problems, fatigue
Vitamin A: Eyes; immune function; skin; essential cell growth and development	Milk, eggs, liver, fortified cereals, orange or green vegetables, fruits	Night blindness, immune function, zinc deficiency, fat malabsorption
Vitamin C: Enzyme activation; second messenger roles (transmitting hormonal information); blood clotting; cell and cell organelle membrane function; nerve impulse transmission and muscular contraction; tone and irritability	Supplementation, broccoli, Brussels sprouts, cantaloupe, cauliflower, citrus, guava, kiwi, papaya, parsley, peas, potatoes, peppers, parsley, rose hips, strawberries, tomatoes	Muscular and nervous irritability, muscle spasms, muscle cramps and tetany, tooth decay, periodontal disease, depression, possibly hypertension

Nutrient/Function	Where It Is Found	Deficiency Symptoms/ Problems
Vitamin D: Calcium and phosphorus levels; calcium absorption; bone mineralization	Sunlight, milk, egg yolks, liver, fish	Osteoporosis, lack of calcium absorption, thyroid disorders, high blood pressure, Parkinson's disease, tuberculosis, cancer, periodontal disease, multiple sclerosis, chronic pain, seasonal affective disorder, peripheral artery disease, cognitive impairment (which includes memory loss and foggy brain), several autoimmune diseases (including type 1 diabetes)
Vitamin K: Aids in formation of clotting factors and bone proteins, formation of glucose into glycogen for storage in the liver	Kale, green tea, turnip greens, spinach, broccoli, lettuce, cabbage, beef liver, asparagus, watercress, cheese, oats, peas, whole wheat	Excessive bleeding, history of bruising, appearance of ruptured capillaries, menorrhagia (heavy periods)

(Information in this chart provided by SpectraCell Laboratories, Inc. Visit: www.spectracell.com)

Prescription medications come with side effects, and all too often these side effects are treated with more medications. Being overmedicated is a common problem in America, especially among the elderly and chronically ill. While medications may be indicated for particular medical conditions, patients need to have a full understanding of the potential side effects.

Micronutrient deficiencies are often a side effect of taking certain prescription medications. If left untreated, the very prescription that was meant for treatment may cause even more health problems. While we can't list all of the medication/deficiency combinations, the most common are listed below.

Drug-Related Micronutrient Deficiency Chart

Drug Type	Drug Name	Associated Common Deficiencies
Antacids/Ulcer Medications	Pepcid®, Tagamet®, Zantac®, Prevacid®, Prilosec®, magnesium and aluminum antacids	Vitamin B12, folic acid, vitamin D, calcium, iron, zinc
Antibiotics	Gentamicin, neomycin, streptomycin, cephalosporins, penicillins, tetracyclines	B vitamins, vitamin K, calcium, magnesium, iron, vitamin B6, zinc
Cholesterol Drugs	Lipitor®, Crestor®, Elavil®, Pamelor®, and others	CoQ10
Antidepressants	Adapin®, Aventyl®, Elavil®, Pamelor®, and others; major tranquilizers (thorazine, Mellaril®, Prolixin®, Serentil®, and others)	CoQ10, vitamin B2
Female Hormones	Estrogen/hormone replacement, oral contraceptives	Vitamin B6, folic acid, vitamin B1, vitamin B2, vitamin B3, vitamin B6, vitamin B12, vitamin C, magnesium, selenium, zinc
Anticonvulsants	Phenobarbital and barbiturates, Dilantin®, Tegretol®, Mysoline®, Depakene®/Depacon®	Vitamin D, calcium, folic acid, biotin, carnitine, vitamin B12, vitamin B1, vitamin K, copper, selenium, zinc
Anti-inflammatories	Steroids: prednisone, Medrol®, Aristocort®, Decadron® NSAIDS (Motrin®, Aleve®, Advil®, Anaprox®, Dolobid®, Feldene®, Naprosyn®, and others) Aspirin and salicylates	Calcium, vitamin D, magnesium, zinc, vitamin C, vitamin B6, vitamin B12, folic acid, selenium, chromium, vitamin C, calcium, iron, vitamin B5

Drug Type	Drug Name	Associated Common Deficiencies
Diuretics	Loop diuretics (Lasix®, Bumex®, Edecrin®), thiazide diuretics (HCTZ, Enduron®, Diuril®, Lozol®, Zaroxolyn®, Hygroton®, and others) Potassium-sparing diuretics	Calcium, magnesium, vitamin B1, vitamin B6, vitamin C, zinc, CoQ10, potassium, folic acid
Cardiovascular Drugs	Antihypertensives (Catapres®, Aldomet®) ACE inhibitors (Capoten®, Vasotec®, Monopril®, and others) Beta blockers (Inderal®, Corgard®, Lopressor®, and others)	CoQ10, vitamin B6, zinc, vitamin B1 Zinc CoQ10
Diabetic Drugs	Metformin® Sulfonylureas (Tolinase®, Micronase®/Glynase®/DiaBeta®),	CoQ10, vitamin B12, folic acid CoQ10
Antiviral Agents	zidovudine (Retrovir®, azidothymidine (AZT), and others) Foscarnet®	Carnitine, copper, zinc, vitamin B12 Calcium, magnesium, potassium

(Information in this chart provided by SpectraCell Laboratories, Inc. Visit www.SpectraCell.com)

Why is it that some people take supplements and still have deficiencies? This may come as a surprise, but the FDA does not regulate supplements. Most store-brand supplements are manufactured in high quantities with little oversight. This lack of quality assurance accounts for the ongoing controversy over supplements and their health benefits, and is the exact reason that we launched our own brand of pharmaceutical-grade supplements (www.stayyoungvitamins.com).

We've had countless patients come in, bags of so-called well-respected supplements in tow, yet they have nothing but abnormal micronutrient test results to show for their lost dollars and time. Do we agree that most supplements are pointless? Yes, we do—not because people don't need the nutritional benefits, but because most of what they are able to purchase is worthless. We feel strongly that supplements should be held to the same standard as other products we put in our bodies, namely food and medicine. Pharmaceutical-grade supplements may cost a bit more, but that's because of the quality ingredients and good manufacturing practices of the laboratories that produce them.

CHAPTER EIGHT

S-E-X

Find the fountain of youth between the sheets

"Sex is a part of nature. I go along with nature" —Marilyn Monroe

Sexuality is a driving force in the lives of humans. Intercourse has multiple health benefits, and a strong libido is a precursor to overall good health. Like the old adage, "If you don't use it, you lose it," sexual interests wane over time if not engaged. Staying active, physically as well as sexually, will increase the chances for a longer life. Sexual intercourse is part of a balanced life, just as vegetables are part of a balanced diet. Our bodies are made to enjoy intercourse as well as reap the benefits of it.

While some believe that sex is reserved for the hormone-raging young adults fresh out of puberty, University of Chicago researchers found that at age 55, most men still have another 15 years of a healthy sex life left, and many have more than that. Actually, men and women well into their 70s and 80s are enjoying sex. According to a recent study of centenarian Cubans, many of them are still enjoying healthy sex lives. While this entire chapter is devoted to the health benefits of sex, we must clarify that monogamous sex has great benefits, but we are not advocating promiscuity, which can lead to a number of health problems, some even fatal.

Little research was done before 1980, but studies in publications such as B. Starr and M. Weiner's *The Starr-Weiner Report on Sex and Sexuality in the Mature Years* (1981) and E. Brecher's *Love, Sex, and Aging* (1984) shed new light on the subject of sex and aging. This research found that there are both physical and emotional benefits to intercourse. These benefits don't diminish with age. Male erections and male and female orgasms can continue throughout life. Of course, this does not mean that they always do. Some medical or psychological issues may limit sexual activity, but nonetheless we are innately wired to be sexual beings.

Men have the ability to produce viable semen for the entirety of life. Ramajit Raghav, a 96-year-old farm laborer in Kharkhoda, Sonipat, is the oldest know man to father a child. Like most lively centenarians, he still gets plenty of exercise, eats a diet high in fresh vegetables, and gets plenty of quality sleep. While it is not our mission to promote parenting at such a late stage in life, it is our mission to encourage people of all ages to have a healthy sex life.

Scientifically, the more sex you have, the higher your levels of pheromones: the scent that makes the opposite sex attracted to you. Imagine your spouse pining after you like they did when you first were newlyweds. Part of that attraction was scientific. To reap the most benefits, we strongly recommend a regimen of sexual intercourse two to three times a week, with strong orgasm.

There are many known health benefits of sex, and studies have shown a strong link between an active sex life and longevity. People are realizing that they are no longer "old" at 50 or 60; therefore, society has been making many adaptations to keep up with sexual desires. As they age, people may seek a younger partner who can meet their biological need. Traditionally, this has been more socially acceptable for men. Recently, though, women are seeking out men that are 10 or 20 years their junior. No longer are relationship parameters constrained by age.

Health Advantages of Sex

Advantage #1: Sex improves cardiovascular health. Sex improves circulation and lowers blood pressure, both of which are extremely important to cardiovascular health. It was once believed that vigorous sex could lead to a heart attack, but research shows that sex twice a week actually reduces the risk of a fatal heart attack. A recent study from Britain researchers found that men who had sex at least twice a week were 45% less likely to have a fatal heart attack than those that had sex less than once a month. Likewise, the act of having sex has no association with increased stroke risk, but instead may actually help prevent it.

Advantage #2: Sex is great exercise. Sex is a great form of exercise. Hitting the sheets three times a week is the equivalent of jogging 75 miles over the course of a year. No time for the gym today? Try "sexercise"—it's a great way to give your rear, legs, and abdominal muscles a great workout.

There are several studies that show the average lovemaking session burns between 50 to 100 calories. That means you could burn 7,500 calories a year just by having sex three times a week. More active sex can increase that caloric burn to as much as 15,000 calories.

"Sex is emotion in motion." —Mae West

Not only is sex good exercise, but exercise outside of sex actually increases sexual desire. Studies have found that those who live sedentary lifestyles, without regular exercise, are more likely to have some sort of sexual dysfunction. Sex and exercise, exercise and sex—the two go hand in hand.

Advantage #3: Sex for brain power. Exercise is a great way to increase memory power. Dr. Brian Christie, a neuroscientist at the University of Victoria in Canada, reports that exercise (like sex) can actually increase your brain size and improve intelligence. Other studies show that sex can decrease the risk of Alzheimer's disease. Sex not only increases blood flow to the brain, it gives the brain a much needed boost of glucose, which can be used as energy. Need a boost in creativity? Sex has long been known to be the inspirational muse to some of the greatest writers and artists.

Advantage #4: Sex for better immunity. Having sex regularly will help fight off colds and the flu. Researchers at Wilkes University in Pennsylvania found that having intercourse 1–2 times a week raises the level of immunoglobin A (IgA), a protein that acts as an antibody by binding to pathogens that enter the body.

Both men and women may receive cancer protection with regular intercourse. A study put out by the National Cancer Institute showed that men may reduce their risk of prostate cancer by as much as one-third by having an orgasm at least three times a week. That study was followed by another at Nottingham University showing that the same regimen could cut the risk of prostate cancer by as much as 50%. Also, the release of DHEA and oxytocin as a result of intercourse gives both men and women protection against breast cancer.

Intercourse has also been shown to heal wounds and stubborn sores. The benefits to the immune system, both known and unknown, affirm that sex is a vital part of our well-being.

Advantage #5: Sex puts a smile on your face. There is no better way to lift your spirits than a little afternoon delight. During sex, mood-boosting hormones are released into the bloodstream. Research shows that these natural hormones reduce anxiety and stress more effectively than prescription sedatives, yet you don't see physicians writing prescriptions for sex (maybe they should). Sex in the morning improves mood, providing a good shot of oxytocin before the business of the day starts.

New research published in 2011 suggests that semen actually has antidepressant qualities. Among the more than 50 components that make up semen, it has many mood-elevating compounds: endorphins, estrone, prolactin, oxytocin, thyrotropin-releasing hormone, and serotonin. These compounds are absorbed vaginally, which further explains the boost in mood for women.

Advantage #6: Sex for better skin and hair. That's right—sex makes you sexy. That post-coital glow is due to the increased blood circulation and increased oxygenation of the blood. Furthermore, orgasms cause a rush of endorphins and growth hormones that repair damaged skin. It also helps the body's natural collagen production, which decreases wrinkles and age spots. A study from researchers in Scotland showed that people who have frequent sex actually look as much as a decade younger than those that don't.

Regular sex increases sex hormones naturally, and also allows the body to absorb nutrients in a more efficient manner. The added benefits of this include strong, healthy hair, skin, and nails.

Advantage #7: Sex as a pain reliever. Oxytocin that is released during orgasm triggers the release of endorphins. Just like prescription pain relievers, these endorphins occupy the pain receptors in the brain and offer relief. So, next time your partner says they have a headache, you can tell them you have the cure.

Advantage #8: Sex for better sleep. The body needs at least 7.5 hours of uninterrupted sleep per night to function at full capacity. Sometimes, getting and staying asleep is hard to do. The oxytocin that is released during sex offers a feeling of contentment, which reduces anxiety and triggers a better night's rest. Regular sex means better sleep, both of which are important to restoring health. If you have the chance for a midday quickie, be sure to leave time for a nap. There is nothing better than a post-coital slumber.

Advantage #9: Sex for a better relationship. Sex is a biological need for both men and women. When people's needs are being met, they are content and easier to get along with. Researchers at the University of Pittsburgh and the University of North Carolina found that couples who have regular sex have higher levels of the "love hormone" oxytocin. This increased their desire to be together and be intimate in ways such as cuddling and holding hands.

A study released in 2012 also suggests that high levels of oxytocin helps keep couples stay monogamous. People having regular sex with their partners are more likely to keep other people of the opposite sex at arm's length. Regular sex is a good form of affair repellent.

Advantage #10: Sex adds years to your life. Multiple studies support that sexual activity and longevity are linked. These findings may be explained by the actual changes in chemistry that take place during intercourse when the body releases dehydroepiandrosterone (DHEA) and human growth hormone (HGH). These hormones maintain youth by assisting in cell and tissue repair. It's no wonder that sex helps you live longer when you consider the cellular changes along with increased circulation, decreased cancer risk, stress reduction, and better sleep.

Researchers at Queens University in Canada who conducted a 10-year study of 1,000 men found that men who had frequent intercourse lived longer than their counterparts who didn't. Next time you're too tired to have sex, remember that your life depends on it.

It's not the number of years but the quality of life one has during those years that is important. Regular sex promotes an active lifestyle at any age—especially in later years. A roll in the hay may prevent a nursing home stay!

Tips for a Better Sex Life

* Enjoy sex with your partner at least three times per week
* Vary the time of day you have sex
* Enjoy sex after a warm shower or bath
* Make weekly date nights a must for your marriage
* Maintain your emotional connection with your partner
* Keep yourself physically fit—this will give you better self-esteem and help your partner stay interested
* Give compliments—if your partner feels good about their body, they are more apt to share it with you
* Learn how to give a good massage and then use that talent at least once a month
* Be conscious of your scent—your body and breath should smell fresh and clean
* Never criticize your partner in bed
* Make sure you kiss during sex—the exchange of saliva is scientifically proven to increase attraction

Lousy Libido?

Libido can change over the years for a number of reasons. It's important to pay attention to your body and recognize when the desire for sex drops off, as this could be indicative of a bigger problem. Because intercourse is a major part of good health, keeping the libido strong is an excellent goal to have. Libido-killers abound, and before you know it, sex drops to the bottom of the priority list. Through education, we can avoid wreaking havoc on one of the best things life has to offer. Thus, what to avoid is covered below.

Smoking. Not only is kissing an ashtray a huge turn-off, smoking can actually damage the blood vessels to the sexual organs. Without adequate blood flow, orgasms become weak or nonexistent.

Sedentary lifestyle. It's time to get up and get moving. Being a couch potato or sitting too long at a desk job can decrease libido and harm overall health. Exercise will improve circulation and increase sex hormone levels naturally.

Weight gain. Drop the extra pounds. Adding a few inches to the waistline will cause hormone fluctuations, something that can send libido into a tailspin. This happens because an increased trunk size decreases the amount of sex hormone–binding globulin (SHBG), which is essential to a healthy sex drive.

Avoid processed carbohydrates. Put down the crackers and cookies. Diets that are high in processed carbohydrates can zap energy levels. It takes energy to have sex, and the more energy, the better the sex. Choose healthy snacks such as fruits and vegetables.

Avoid the "D". Flu and allergy medicines can ruin sex drive. Avoid decongestants, usually marked with a "D" on cold and allergy medications. These ingredients can cause major sexual dysfunction.

Blood pressure medication. This may be the most overlooked problem in men. The same medications that lower blood pressure decrease the blood flow to the genital area. Certain blood pressure medications are worse than others. Talk to your doctor if your medication is keeping down more than just your blood pressure.

Hair growth drugs. Get a transplant or get a hat. Drugs that are intended to help regrow hair, such as finasteride (Proscar®, Propecia®), have an erectile dysfunction rate as high as 92% in its users.

Diabetes. Keep the sugar under control. Diabetics suffer from circulation problems as well as low hormone levels. Even in pre-diabetic states, libido can suffer.

Low testosterone. This is a problem for both sexes: testosterone plays an important role in sexual desire in both men and women. Levels of this hormone can gradually decrease over time. Women who have been on birth control pills for many years will also see a significant drop in testosterone as they reach the second half of their third decade. Bio-identical hormone replacement can be prescribed and monitored by a qualified healthcare provider.

Micronutrient deficiencies. This is an easy thing to fix. Micronutrient deficiencies can cause a lack of libido. For example, a zinc deficiency is a frequent finding in those who suffer from erectile dysfunction, low libido, or depression.

HOWARD HALL, 92 YEARS YOUNG, FRANKFORT, KENTUCKY

Competes in track and field and swimming—has earned over 600 medals in local, state, and National Senior Games since 1987 (Personal Best profile at www.NSGA.com). "Unless you have actual pain or physical impairment, you should always try to do a little more than what you feel like you want to do. Competing in [the] Senior Games has kept me fit. It's a means of making me do my exercises. I don't want to look foolish out there, so it drives me to stay in good shape. I do calisthenics in the morning—pushups and ab crunches. Then I generally walk two miles every morning to get a newspaper, and I will often sprint 100 yards during it. And I try to go swim twice a week, and bowl some too at the Y."

CHAPTER 9

THE BALANCING ACT

Health and your hormones

"The best and safest thing is to keep a balance in your life,
acknowledge the great powers around us and in us. If you can do
that, and live that way, you are really a wise man." —Euripides

---

Hormones define who we are. They are the messengers that govern development in the early years and continue to regulate well-being and metabolism throughout life. Hormone levels have a direct effect on health, personality, and energy. For teenagers, extremely high levels of hormones can cause mood swings, increased sexual interest, and fluctuation in sleep patterns. This is why teens can sometimes stay up for hours, and other times barely get out of bed. Likewise, during pregnancy, hormones cause all kinds of changes to the body, including food cravings, swelling, nausea, forgetfulness, and so on.

When we age, decreases in our hormone levels continue to affect us, causing slower cognition (also known as foggy brain), weight gain, decrease in lean muscle mass, irritability, and changes in the skin and hair. These changes take place in both men and women. To most people's surprise, men and women both have testosterone and estrogen. A balance or imbalance of sex and thyroid hormones is a big factor in defining a person's personality, strength, health, and mental clarity. Defining and understanding hormones is the first step in appreciating the need for balance. The following is a list of some of the major hormones and their functions.

Estrogen. Estradiol is the most common and effective form of estrogen in the body. Both men and women have estradiol, but it plays a larger role in women than it does in men. This hormone is important to bone health, heart health, mood, libido, proper thyroid function, skin elasticity, and blood sugar levels. Women need estrogen in order to reproduce. In the years leading up to and after menopause, the decrease in estradiol levels can cause significant changes, which speed the aging process. Estrogen is also referred to as the feminizing hormone.

In men, estradiol is usually suppressed by testosterone. When testosterone levels drop, the ratio of estradiol to testosterone changes and can cause weight gain, enlarged breasts (gynecomastia), and a loss of sex drive. When it comes to estrogen in men, the ratio of estrogen to testosterone is very important. For men, the ratio should be 20:1—twenty times more testosterone than estrogen. For women, the ratio is more dependent upon symptoms than any given percentage. Balance is key.

Progesterone. Progesterone is found in both sexes and is a precursor to both estrogen and testosterone. In women, progesterone is essential to childbirth. During menopause the level of progesterone decreases, and the deficit can cause a number of menopausal symptoms. Progesterone is not a feminizing hormone, but rather a natural antagonist of estrogen.

In men, changes in progesterone levels are often associated with changes in testosterone levels. Men produce progesterone in their testes and women produce it in the corpus luteum of the ovaries after ovulation. In both men and women, the adrenal glands also produce a small amount of progesterone. Progesterone is important to libido, bone growth, metabolism, thyroid regulation, mood, sleep, and salt metabolism.

Luteinizing hormone (LH). LH is produced in the pituitary gland. For women, this hormone plays a big role in ovulation, which usual occurs mid-cycle. LH also helps stimulate testosterone production in men. Low levels of LH may be a symptom of hypopituitarism. A higher than normal level in women is a sign of menopause or polycystic ovaries. In men, a high level can be associated with hypogonadism.

Follicle-stimulating hormone (FSH). FSH is found in both men and women and is released from the anterior pituitary gland. This hormone is called a gonadotropin because it stimulates the gonads. In women, it stimulates the production of eggs and estradiol, and regulates the menstrual cycle. In men, it stimulates production of sperm. FSH is essential to both puberty and menopause. As women age and reach menopause, FSH levels go up. For healthy males, these levels stay relatively constant as they age. Ovarian failure, testicular failure, pituitary tumors, adrenal, thyroid, or autoimmune diseases can cause FSH levels to fluctuate in an unpredictable manner. This is why changes in hormones should always be evaluated by a physician who has a clear understanding of the endocrine system and the latest research on hormones.

Testosterone. Testosterone is a steroid hormone that is important to both sexes. Women only have 5%–10% of the testosterone that men have, but nevertheless, it is still essential to overall health. Men make testosterone in their testes and women make it in their ovaries. Both sexes make a small amount in the adrenal glands.

Testosterone plays a crucial role in stimulating muscle and bone growth, maintaining adequate energy levels, regulating mood, retaining electrolytes, and promoting a healthy sexual desire. Testosterone is important to heart health and the prevention of Alzheimer's disease. It also protects against breast cancer and prostate cancer.

A decrease in testosterone can cause a number of symptoms, including loss of lean muscle mass and increase in fat, loss of mental clarity, loss of ambition and stamina, moodiness, low energy levels, and a decrease in sex drive. A deficiency can have these negative effects on both men and women alike.

About the Thyroid

Generally weighing less than one ounce, it's hard to believe that such a small gland could have so much power. The thyroid gland is located in the front of the neck just below the Adam's apple and is shaped like a butterfly. It is controlled by the pituitary, a peanut-sized gland located at the base of the brain. The thyroid gland is the body's furnace, and that pituitary gland is the thermostat that controls its activity.

The thyroid is the only gland that has the ability to absorb iodine, taking it in and converting it to thryroxine (T4) and triiodothyronine (T3). Every cell in the body is dependent upon thyroid hormones for its metabolic process. That is why an imbalance of thyroid hormones can wreak havoc on the body, causing all types of unwelcome symptoms.

Sometimes, poor nutrition, medications, or life circumstances can inhibit the thyroid from functioning properly. Nutrients such as iron, iodine, selenium, zinc, and riboflavin, and vitamins A and B12, are all important to normal thyroid function. Medications such as birth control pills and beta blockers can inhibit the conversion of T4 to T3, a necessary process in thyroid hormone balance. Even stress, surgical procedures, and alcohol can have a negative effect on these hormones.

Thyroid hormones regulate temperature, weight, heart rhythm, energy levels, hair health, and appetite. Even the slightest change in these hormones can have outward signs and symptoms.

Triiodothyronine (T3). T3 comprises only 20% of the total hormones released by the thyroid, but has four times the power of T4. T3 plays a major role in metabolism. Low levels could suggest an underactive thyroid gland, and high levels, an overactive one.

Thyroxine (T4). T4 is more abundant and makes up 80% of the thyroid hormones; however, it is inactive. It is called T4 because it contains four iodine atoms. T4 comes in two forms: one that is attached to proteins and prevented from entering cells, and free T4 (FT4), which can enter targeted tissues and aid with metabolism. T3 is the more useful form of the two, so T4 must lose one of its iodine atoms to convert to T3.

Thyroid-stimulating hormone (TSH). Controlled by the pituitary gland, TSH is released when T3 and T4 drop below optimal levels. TSH stimulates the thyroid to produce more T3 and T4 and send it into the bloodstream. This level can be confusing because it seems backward. A high TSH means that the thyroid is underactive, and a low TSH is a sign of overactivity.

Cortisol. Cortisol is a steroid hormone that is secreted by the adrenal gland. In normal amounts, cortisol can help the body react to stress and environmental changes. When the body has a "fight-or-flight" response, cortisol is released and allows the body to react appropriately. Cortisol levels should fluctuate during the day, with the highest levels occurring in the morning. When cortisol levels remain at a constant high level due to chronic stress, the body will react negatively. High levels of cortisol can artificially suppress TSH, affect blood sugar, raise blood pressure, cause weight gain, and lower immunity.

Hormones and Age

As we age, hormone levels change dramatically. Hormone levels should be monitored yearly, and for those who qualify, hormone replacement therapy may be a great option. There are many types of hormone replacement therapies, and the right type and combination depend on individual needs. When managed properly, hormone replacement therapy can lead to a healthy and active life filled with energy and vigor.

When Hormone Replacement Therapy Is NOT a Fit

While hormone replacement therapy can be a great way for some people to stay feeling youthful, it's not for everybody. Certain medical conditions will disqualify someone from receiving hormones, because they could cause undesirable side effects. Be sure to discuss your medical history with your physician prior to starting any type of hormone replacement. Below is a list of disqualifiers:

Women with a history of breast, uterine, ovarian, or cervical cancer[2]

Women with undiagnosed vaginal bleeding

Men with a history of prostate cancer within the last five years

Men with a *prostate-specific antigen* (PSA) over 2.5 who have not been cleared with a full urological work-up to rule out the possibility of prostate cancer

Both men and women with a history of mental conditions, such as bipolar disorder, borderline personality disorder, or anxiety neurosis

Synthetic hormone replacement therapy. Synthetic hormones are hormones that have been made in a laboratory through synthetic means. These hormones started from natural sources (plants and animals), but in order to have the body metabolize them, they were chemically changed. Therefore, they are close, but not identical, to the hormones produced by the body. While synthetic hormones may help with symptoms of menopause or erectile dysfunction, in some cases, they have been associated with unwanted side effects.

Bio-identical hormone replacement therapy (BHRT). Made from natural plant sources, such as soy and yam, bio-identical hormones are professionally compounded

---

[2] This only applies to estrogen and progesterone, and does not affect candidacy for testosterone replacement.

by a compounding pharmacist to be bio-identical to the forms of estrogen and testosterone that are found in the human body. This allows the body to utilize them as if it has produced them itself. The use of bio-identical hormones is experiencing a surge in popularity in North America, but they have been studied and used effectively in Europe for decades.

Bio-identical hormones come in different forms, such as creams and pellets. Both have advantages and disadvantages. The creams are an easy way to apply BHRT, and are preferred by those who may not be able to get to the physician for implants every three to six months. Some of the downsides of using a cream include fluctuating levels during the day, the notion that they are inconvenient for travel, and that there is a risk of absorption by loved ones and pets. Pellets, another option, are inserted just under the skin in the buttock area and dissolve at a continuous rate. They last anywhere from three to six months and then must be replaced. The disadvantage to pellets is that once they are in, they stay in until they dissolve on their own. In almost all cases, this is not a problem. If need be, the amount and frequency of the BHRT can be changed over time according to symptoms and/or absorption rates.

Bio-identical pellet therapy should always come from a reputable source. These pellets are made at compounding pharmacies, and not all pellets are manufactured the same. We prefer to obtain our pellets from BioTE Medical—not only because they have a proven track record, but because in our experience they have a dosing system that delivers less side effects and greater efficacy.

Prior to hormone replacement therapy, a number of laboratory and diagnostic tests must be completed. This will ensure that the replacement dose is correctly calculated, and will also give the physician a clearer picture of the patient's health status. In some cases, abnormal results may be an indication for further investigation or disqualification from BHRT. These tests include:

Complete blood count
Comprehensive metabolic panel
Estradiol
Free T3
Free testosterone (males only)

FSH
Hemoglobin A1C
PSA (males only)
Total testosterone
TSH
Vitamin B12
Vitamin D 25-hydroxy
Other labs as suggested[3]

What Sparks the Flame and What Keeps It Going

For years, people have attributed good relationships to "great chemistry." Long before the science of attraction was discovered, people understood that something within the body changes when love is on the horizon. From love (or lust) at first sight to a life-long commitment, hormones play a big role. Just like the song suggests, this explains how people can become addicted to love.

First Moment of Attraction: The stage when flirting occurs. Testosterone and estrogen levels increase, and often the body puts off pheromones.

Romantic Love: Most recognizable by the constant mood swings. Romantic love includes moments of euphoria when together, followed by despair when separated. A simple fight may feel like the end of the world. The hormones in this phase can bring about physical symptoms as well, including sweaty palms, butterflies in the stomach, weight loss, and lack of sleep. The culprits include a number of hormones, all flooding the system and creating chaos throughout the body.

1   DOPAMINE is mostly associated with the feeling of pleasure. The feeling it brings to the body causes a natural form of reinforcement. Dopamine release is often found with physical intimacy.

2   PHENYLETHYLAMINE is a natural amphetamine that is released during romantic love. This is what gives that sense of "high" and allows people to stay up all

---

[3] Because hormone levels can also be affected by micronutrient deficiencies, we strongly encourage patients to have a micronutrient test, reviewing 26 different nutrient levels, prior to BHRT. Correcting deficiencies can increase the absorption and utilization of the hormones being replaced.

hours of the night just so they can spend more time together.

3   SEROTONIN helps to control impulses and obsessive behavior. This keeps the relationship on track and moving in the right direction.

4   NOREPINEPHRINE is responsible for the raised blood pressure and pounding of the heart when a lover is present. It's a natural adrenaline booster, and induces the feeling of euphoria.

The Long Haul: What keeps the flame burning. A sense of responsibility may be a good start to a long-lasting relationship, but the hormones behind lasting love are the glue that bind. The hormones that give the feelings of calmness and stability are what keep couples together. Some of these hormones also act as a shield against infidelity.

5   OXYTOCIN influences our ability to bond with one another. Both genders release this hormone when they touch each other or cuddle together. Oxytocin levels peak during orgasm, creating a bond and promoting monogamy.

6   VASOPRESSIN is another chemical that helps with fidelity. Researchers discovered that the suppression of vasopressin can lead to males leaving the relationship. Praise and love help raise vasopressin, while conflict and criticism suppress it.

7   ENDORPHINS help lower stress and improve memory. They also calm anxiety and give the body a sense of attachment and comfort with its partner.

Understanding the symptoms of hormone deficiencies and imbalance will significantly reduce the chance of misdiagnosis. Patients need to be empowered with knowledge so they can relay information to their healthcare provider accurately and fully. For example, if a patient just complains of depressive symptoms during an exam, they may be put on antidepressants. However, if a patient explains *all* the symptoms they are having, hormone levels will more likely be checked.

Common symptoms in men with hormone deficiencies or imbalance:

* Decreased sex drive
* Erectile dysfunction
* Muscle loss
* Osteoporosis
* Weight gain

- Increased body fat
- Breast enlargement
- Memory loss
- Irritability
- Depression
- Restless sleep
- Fatigue
- Bladder weakness
- Blood sugar imbalance
- Cholesterol imbalance
- Excessive sweating

Common symptoms in women with hormone deficiencies or imbalance:

- Irregular periods
- Weight gain
- Hot flashes
- Mood swings
- Loss of energy
- Decreased strength
- Increased abdominal fat
- Joint pain
- Osteoporosis
- Irritability
- Brain fog
- Loss of sex drive
- Vaginal dryness
- Night sweats
- Headaches

* Restless sleep
* Loss of breast fullness
* Depression

Common improvements experienced with bio-identical hormone optimization:

* Improves mental function and clarity
* Relieves anxiety
* Reduces depressive symptoms
* Increases metabolism
* Restores sexual function and increases libido
* Reduces or eliminates hormone-triggered migraines
* Builds lean muscle mass
* Reduces excess fat around the midline
* Decreases or eliminates menopausal symptoms, such as hot flashes, night sweats, and insomnia

As you can see from the lists above, hormones are not just about libido. They play a big role in overall health. As the chronological clock ticks, the levels of hormones decline and so does the body. Taking time to have hormones assessed and optimized may dramatically improve quality of life.

CHAPTER 10

THE 3'S OF EXERCISE

Three types, 30 minutes, three times a week

> "My grandmother started walking five miles a day when she was 60. She's 97 now, and we don't know where the heck she is." —Ellen DeGeneres

While recent medical advancements allow us to save more lives than ever before, modern technology as a whole has lessened our level of activity. Modern conveniences allow many of us to meet our needs with very little physical activity. Americans have a higher obesity rate than at any other time in history, partially due to the change in the work environment. Most jobs are no longer physically taxing, and sitting for long periods of time is common in the workplace.

When we researched and interviewed those that have lived long and relatively healthy lives, there was a common thread among all of them. They had many years of physical activity and manual labor. This level of activity was necessary for survival, and most didn't mind because they had never been exposed to an alternative. Exercise was just a part of life, not something that was scheduled for recreational purposes.

Today, we have to make an effort to get the proper amount of exercise. Sometimes, going to the gym is just too much of an inconvenience and falls to the bottom of the priority list, which is a mistake. Exercise should always be a high priority. In addition, finding the time is only part of the equation. The type of exercise you do and how long you do it matters.

Most of our patients claim that they get enough exercise, but their records and health say otherwise. Some may be doing a little of this and a little of that, but they haven't really committed to regular exercise program. Getting in shape doesn't require a fancy trainer or expensive club membership. A good workout requires only what is readily available: the floor, walls, and body weight.

The 3 Types

Exercise can be divided into three different types: cardiovascular, muscle building, and flexibility. All three are important to help the body maintain strength and avoid injury. Each type of exercise has its own benefits, and when all are incorporated into a regular regimen, total fitness can be achieved.

Cardiovascular exercise, also referred to as aerobic exercise, is achieved when the heart and lungs are being challenged. Some examples of cardiovascular exercise include running, elliptical training, swimming, and dancing. During this type of exercise, the lungs expand fully, maximizing the amount of oxygen in the blood. As the heart beats faster, circulation is improved throughout the body. Cardio exercise is critical to the detoxification process because it allows the small blood vessels (capillaries) to widen. This widening facilitates the flow of waste away from different parts of the body, preparing it to be discarded.

"Get comfortable with being uncomfortable!" —Jillian Michaels

Muscle building is for everyone, not just for those that want to gain bulk. Muscles, especially the core and large muscle groups, need resistance to stay healthy. Not only can this type of exercise be done by lifting weights, it can also be done by using one's own body weight—for example, with push-ups or chin-ups. Muscle building is important because it helps improve metabolism: lean muscle mass burns more calories than a flabby set of muscles, and it takes more energy to support muscle than fat. The American College of Sports Medicine (ACSM) recommends 10 strength-training exercises, with 8–12 repetitions. This should be done twice a week with several days between training so the muscles have time to repair.

Flexibility exercises are often overlooked when planning a fitness regimen. Remaining flexible will help prevent injuries as well as prevent arthritis. George Burns, one of the world's most famous centenarians, was no stranger to exercise. He also maintained unbelievable flexibility—he was still able to touch his toes into his last and final decade of life. The simple act of stretching increases blood supply and delivers vital nutrients to joint structures. That's why stretching is often referred to as warming up: it raises the body temperature around the joints. Synovial fluid, the fluid that lubricates the joints, is increased with stretching. More fluid means healthier joints, less arthritis, and less pain. Flexibility exercises increase range of motion and help prevent injury and joint degeneration.

30 Minutes or More

Most people think they get enough exercise, but when they actually start writing down how much time they spend sitting as opposed to exercising, they are shocked. It doesn't take much exercise to make a significant difference in health. And, it's a matter of being consistent. A Danish study that was published in the *American Journal of Physiology* reported that 30 minutes of exercise is just as effective as a full hour. While the study was about weight loss and body composition, it would make sense that the overall health benefits would follow suit.

How your exercise time is spent can change throughout the week. For example, one day can be 20 minutes of cardiovascular, followed by muscle building. The next day of exercise can be yoga. Changing up the exercise routine will keep it from getting mundane and prevent a loss of interest. When exercising for 30 minutes, remember that the timer doesn't start until the actual exercise does.

3 Times a Week

Exercising a minimum of three times a week will help you reap the benefits listed later in this chapter. If you can squeeze in five times, that's even better. Marking the calendar with workout days will help it become engrained in your daily routine. For example: set aside Monday, Thursday, and Saturday (or any other days) for your scheduled workouts. Anything squeezed in during other days is a bonus.

Motivation for working out is all about attitude. If someone sees exercise as "me" time and understands that it has a number of benefits, they are more likely to keep up a regular routine. Once exercise becomes a chore or just one more thing to accomplish for the day, exercise is less likely to happen.

The best way to keep a schedule and stick to it is to have an exercise partner, someone who will commit to it. When two or more people are involved, exercise becomes as much as a social activity as it is a necessity. It also takes the intimidation factor out of going to an exercise class or joining a gym. Frankly, working out with a friend can be great therapy, too. Some of the biggest problems have been solved while running around a track. In 1993, President Bill Clinton put a jogging track next to the White House and used it to gain perspective each morning.

TOP 20 BENEFITS OF EXERCISE

1 Reach or maintain a healthy body weight
2 Improve immunity and ward off colds and other illnesses
3 Increase energy levels and prevent fatigue
4 Prevent depression and control anxiety
5 Prevent some cancers and improve ability to recover from others
6 Reduce the risk of osteoporosis
7 Keep blood pressure and pulse rates low
8 Maintain normal blood sugar levels, preventing diabetes
9 Increase circulation
10 Clear the body of toxins that can cause pain and physiological stress on the body
11 Improve and stabilize hormone levels
12 Improve memory and cognitive skills
13 Lower cholesterol
14 Improve relationships through improved mood
15 Increase the chances of living independently in later years
16 Increased longevity
17 Relief from pain caused by migraines, menstrual cramps, or arthritis
18 Improved libido and sexual function
19 Improved sleep quality
20 Improved metabolism

In addition to a regular exercise routine, making little changes in lifestyle will also increase overall mobility. It's the small, everyday changes that add up. If you adopt each suggestion on the list below, your activity level will change significantly in a matter of a month, and you're likely to drop a few pounds. Exercise begets more exercise, so the more you move, the more your body will encourage you to move. A sedentary lifestyle can be turned around—even if you have never been a fan of exercise.

> "You've got to keep your body active, even if that means just turning on some music and dancing for an hour... That's how you'll prepare your bodies and your minds for greatness." —Michelle Obama

Choose a parking spot that is far from the entry to the store. This is a great way to add a few steps to your day.

- When you have the choice, take the stairs and skip the elevator.
- Take five-minute breaks at work and stretch. This will help increase blood flow and stimulate tired muscles.
- Pick either the morning or evening, but walk your neighborhood block at least three days a week.
- When your car is dirty, wash it by hand. This is a great way to incorporate all the components of a good workout into a 30- to 45-minute session.
- Do 20 jumping jacks a day for a week, then add 10 more each week until you reach 100 per day.
- Have sex three times a week. Consider it exercise with benefits, or sexercise.

Out of all the prescriptions we write, exercise is the most important. If you follow a regular exercise regimen based on the principles above, many other prescriptions will never need to be written. Not only will this save you money, it will also eliminate unnecessary side effects. A strong body is a body that is built to last.

JOHN TATUM, 94 YEARS YOUNG, WASHINGTON, D.C.

Swimmer who has competed in National Senior Games since 2003, won three gold medals in each of the past two games (Personal Best profile at www.NSGA. com). "What I tell people first is to take care of your body. I tell them to exercise, keep going. I like to swim for exercise mostly, but it's been fun to do these races, too. I swim three times a week, and enjoy competing and the camaraderie of my team. I've also been gardening for probably 50 years now. You have to keep moving. That's what it's all about."

CHAPTER ELEVEN

THE FUTURE OF MEDICINE

DNA, personalized medicine, and stem cells

"DNA is like a computer program but far, far more advanced than any software ever created." —Bill Gates, *The Road Ahead*

When Watson and Crick discovered the double-helix structure of DNA in 1953, it seemed as if all the secrets of human existence had been realized. As we now know, that discovery was but the first step in a journey that is still unfolding to this day. The nature of medicine is much like a Pandora's box, with each new discovery leading to another. Some new truth about life, our existence, and our future is being realized even as you are reading the words on this page.

Physicians practicing today will tell you that medicine moves at a pace that's hard for even the most advanced healthcare providers to keep up with. There are new drugs coming to market almost daily. Each year sees the introduction of more advanced, efficient treatment techniques. New discoveries have the ability to completely alter our concept of the same familiar disease we have been treating for years. But at this moment in time, we are on the cusp of a completely new way of looking at medicine as a whole. What healthcare providers are taught about disease, prevention, and treatment is all being changed by a discovery that started 60 years ago. Even the things taught in the next five to 10 years will pale in comparison to where we will be 50 years from today. We are embarking on what we like to call…Generation Genetics!

Personal Genetic Testing

Once the Human Genome Project was complete, the Personal Genome Project began, recognizing that each person is unique and that the future of health and medicine is not a one-size-fits-all recipe. Personal genetic testing has taken hold around the world and is being embraced by private companies, educational institutions, and even some governments.

"And now the announcement of Watson and Crick about DNA. This is for me the real proof of the existence of God." —Salvador Dali

---

In the United Kingdom, people are lining up to donate their DNA and medical records to help unlock the secrets that some day may save their children or grandchildren. Their national government is backing this 500,000-person study. By studying subjects aged 40–69, this study will improve the wait time for answers to diabetes, heart disease, and cancer, because this is the age group that these diseases are most prevalent in.

Personal genomics is here to stay. Stanford University added personal genotyping to their curriculum with the Genetics 210: Genomics and Personalized Medicine course, where students are able to learn using their own genetic information. It was the university's belief, and we agree, that medical students are more likely to dig deeper and learn more if they can incorporate their own genetic information into the subject they are studying. Today's medical students and young scientists will carry forth the torch of medicine, saving lives in larger numbers than ever before.

Desperately
Needing
Answers

A personal reflection...

Personal genetic sequencing is mired in a variety of ethical questions. There are concerns, for example, about how people may respond to learning they are predisposed to a given disease. I remember reading the consents prior to sending my DNA to 23andMe for sequencing. I almost turned back, harkened by the siren song "ignorance is bliss." Then I thought about my spouse and my children. I had to ask myself these questions: Would I look back someday and wish I had a clue? Would the information guide me to make better lifestyle choices? The answer to both was a definite YES.

Once my DNA sequencing data was back, I realized that I had an increased risk for Alzheimer's, something that I had already suspected. I also learned that I was not genetically disposed to multiple sclerosis or colon cancer, both of which are in my family history. Maybe the most surprising finding was that I carry the genetic code for cystic fibrosis. Luckily, I hadn't married another carrier—this could have put my children at risk for developing the disease and possibly dying at a very young age. After this discovery, two of my daughters who are over the age of 18 had their DNA sequenced. One of them was a carrier and the other was not.

My reason for sharing this information with you, the reader, is to help shed light on the purpose of personal DNA sequencing. It should be done in the right frame of mind, within the right context, and with the right purpose. I was well informed of the potential risks for discovering what may or may not be my future. I know that just because I have a predisposition, it is not a guarantee of disease, and I can do my part to prevent that specific gene from ever being expressed.

The testing did not make me feel trapped—quite the contrary. I felt freed by the information because it helped me stay in the driver's seat of my health and my life. I was able to have real and informed conversations with my children about my predispositions and how it relates to them and their future. As far as the Alzheimer's gene, I made a pact with my family, asking them now while I am of sound mind, to start treatment early, even if I am in denial. No regrets, no squabbling, and no guilt. My wishes for my life.

DNA sequencing is not for everyone. If you choose to have your DNA sequenced, please be sure to do it with clear thought and mind. Be informed about all that it involves and make the most out of your results.

—Judy Gaman

Personalized Medicine

In the near future, personal DNA will be just another part of the medical record. Just like a person's individual medical history and family history can tell a story about the past, personal DNA may give clues to the future. Imagine going to the doctor and getting the right treatment the first time and averting what could have been a dangerous allergic reaction. Finding out this way is a vast improvement over the old way. Personalized medicine will soon take the guesswork out of treatments.

Pharmacogenomics is the study of how certain medications and diseases interface with genetic variations. Technology is already available to identify people who may not respond to cholesterol-lowering medicines, or could have harmful reactions to certain blood thinners. Perhaps one of the widest and most significant uses of pharmacogenomics is in cancer treatment, which can now be highly personalized based on the person's biological makeup.

The unlocking of personal genomes will continue to change the way patients are treated. With a way to narrow down research and development efforts, medical treatments are destined to be more effective and more efficient than ever before.

Nanobots

With the new technology of nanobots, engineering and medicine collide. This tiny little discovery, also referred to as nanites or nanomachines, are by definition equal to one-billionth of one meter, or the width of 10 atoms. These very small robots enter the body to complete specific tasks, such as repair damaged tissue. While they are only in the early stages of development, hope is that they will be able to be programmed to enter the body with a specific mission and repair bad cells without harm to healthy cells. For example, nanobots may someday be able to enter the body to identify cancerous cells, wiping them out while leaving the tissue around them virtually untouched.

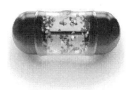

In 1989, IBM was the first to prove that individual atoms could be manipulated, a discovery that was a precursor to nanotechnology. With the mid-to-late 2020s being the target for the use of nanotechnology in medicine, it's hard to believe that this much advancement could happen in a span of just 30-plus years.

Stem Cells for a Brighter Future

Academic institutions around the globe have joined forces to change the face of medicine forever. The University of Wisconsin–Madison uncovered that stem cells may be the answer to neurological disorders such as ALS, Parkinson's disease, epilepsy, and stroke. Their research has proven that human embryonic stem cells, when transplanted into the brain of mice, can send and receive nerve impulses.

Scientists at Northwestern University in Illinois have used embryonic stem cells to make neurons, the same cells found in the brain. By adding chemical growth factors to the human embryonic stem cells, scientists are now able to grow a nearly unlimited supply of brain cells. This discovery is likely to play a big role in the research and development of future Alzheimer's medications, as well as pave the way for neuron transplants.

> "The problem [with genetic research] is, we're just starting down this path, feeling our way in the dark. We have a small lantern in the form of a gene, but the lantern doesn't penetrate more than a couple of hundred feet. We don't know whether we're going to encounter chasms, rock walls or mountain ranges along the way. We don't even know how long the path is." —Francis S. Collins

Some scientists are even working with Wellcome Trust in Great Britain with the goal of forming a synthetic form of O-negative blood through the use of stem cells. A discovery like this could prove to be invaluable during times of war or natural disasters.

The advancements in stem cell research are unending, covering areas that range from cancer vaccinations to a cure for diabetes. It seems that scientists around the world have all embraced the possibilities. For example, scientists in Singapore and Japan are working hard to develop stem cell solutions to heart disease.

During the research for this book, we had the distinct pleasure of visiting International Stem Cell Corporation (ISCO) in California. This publicly traded biotechnology company is devoted to regenerative medicine through ethical means. Spending a day with these bright minds was a very humbling experience and one we will never forget. The scientists work tirelessly for the purpose of helping others have a brighter future.

ISCO uses a new technology called parthenogenesis. Since partheno means "virgin" and genesis means "birth," it's a fitting name for stem cell research that uses unfertilized human eggs that can be immune-matched to millions of people, regardless of sex or race. Their research may represent the greatest breakthrough of all because it does not involve embryos, thus avoiding the ethical objections that have held back so much research in the past. While at the lab, we witnessed the great work they are doing with reference to the eye, nervous system, and liver. The development of a human cornea made directly from the technology they have worked so hard to develop was especially intriguing.

Stem Cells for a Younger-Looking You

The same stem cell research that ISCO is using toward regenerative medicine can actually help turn back the effects of time on the skin. Lifeline Skin Care, a division of ISCO, has developed a non-embryonic human stem cell extract serum that helps regenerate the skin, especially the face, neck and hands, where people show the most aging. The best part about this product is that a portion of the proceeds from the serum sales go toward funding other life-changing research that ISCO is undertaking.

We have seen great results with Lifeline®, not only with ourselves, but with so many of our patients. This line of stem cell creams has transformed skin, erasing wrinkles, dark spots, and old acne scars. The creams can be ordered at www.stayyoungskin.com.

The secrets to living a long and healthy life, really aren't secrets at all. Even as we unveil new information about humans and the world around us, good health practices remain the same: eat right, exercise on a regular basis, get adequate sleep, and keep stress levels to a minimum. Through all the medical breakthroughs of the past and all those to come, truth will remain truth. Regardless of what the future holds, good health always starts with the present.

BILL MEAGHER, 93 YEARS YOUNG, VIRGINIA BEACH, VIRGINIA

Life is an exciting journey for Bill. His greatest adventure: serving as Navigator aboard the USS *Mount Olympus,* flagship for the Navy's Operation "High Jump," the famous 1946 Antarctic expedition led by Adm. Richard E. Byrd. "Do the hard things first, then everything else is easy!"

CHAPTER TWELVE

WORDS FROM THE WISE

Advice from living centenarians

"Young. Old. Just words" —George Burns

The best way to create a book about living to 100 is to include advice straight from the mouths of those who have actually "been there and done that." Since they have 10 decades to their credit, they actually lived through what most people only read about in history books. Next time you feel overwhelmed by the evening news, frustrated with a deadline at work, or angry toward someone who offends you, take time to put it into perspective. Most things are but a speck of ink on the pages that fill our lives.

Centenarians remember firsthand both World Wars, the sinking of the Titanic, Albert Einstein winning the Nobel Prize, Charles Lindbergh's first flight, the erection of the Empire State Building, the rise and fall of Hitler, the Great Depression, the attack on Pearl Harbor, detonation of atomic bombs, the Korean War, the first man in space, the construction and destruction of the Berlin Wall, the Vietnam War, the assassination of one president and resignation of another, Chernobyl, two Gulf Wars, and much more. They were born into a world driven mostly by horse and buggy, without indoor plumbing, television, or any of today's conveniences. This generation communicated without the use of computers or cell phones, and they received news through word of mouth and print. The Internet and CNN would have sounded like the musings of a mad man. However, day by day, things progressed.

This generation adapted quite well as the world around them changed at a phenomenally fast pace. Almost everything they once knew has changed, but regardless of how the world evolves, the human spirit remains the same. The following is a glimpse into the most resilient generation, one that holds a wealth of information and wisdom that most of us can't even begin to comprehend. May their stories inspire you and bring a new understanding of what it means to actually live and do it well.

Four Hundred Years of Good, Sound Advice

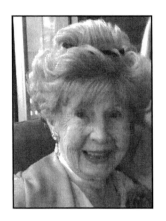

Lucille Fleming, 100 years and 6 months, Bedford, Texas
Maybe one of the most inspiring individuals we have ever had the pleasure of meeting, Lucille is what we lovingly refer to as a "firecracker." Originally from Canada, she traveled to the United States at the ripe age of 17. After earning enough money to put herself through college, she studied to be a nurse and went on to work at Massachusetts General. She is no stranger to longevity; her mother lived to be 96, her father 92, and she had a maternal uncle that reached 99. Lucille suffered a broken femur in 1994. This misfortune would have led most down a path of demise, but for her it was just a small bump in the road. Her elegant, well-decorated apartment is an indication of her continued independence. It has a full kitchen and a living room for entertaining her guests, something she does quite often.

Quite frankly, she has better overall cognitive skills and memory than most of the patients we see every day, many of whom are 50 or 60 years her junior. When asked about her daily routine, she responded with the following:

"My breakfast consists of oatmeal, strawberries, and cottage cheese. I have enjoyed fresh fruits and vegetables from the garden since I was a small child. One of my favorite fruits is blueberries, which I have always enjoyed in fairly large quantities. I brush my teeth three times a day, but never been one for flossing."

"I say my prayers in the morning when rising and at night before going to bed. I'm thankful for each day and glad to know where I am and who I am."

When asked for her top ten tips for making it to 100-plus, here is what she provided us:

1. Look at the bright side of things and be happy.

2. Eat a good diet. Three times a day, be sure to get in fresh fruits and vegetables.

3. Exercise every day. While I used to walk six miles a day, I still get in a little over a half a mile.

4. Be social. Have many friends and spend time with them. My father never knew a stranger and invited everyone that pulled up in their horse and buggy to come in for dinner. I like to be social by playing double bridge because it keeps the mind sharp.

5. Work crossword puzzles and read. I have macular degeneration, but that doesn't stop me. I just deal with it.

6. Take an interest in things. I love to watch the Dallas Cowboys, the Texas Rangers, and political debates.

7. If you have a religion, go to church.

8. Spend time with family. If you have an issue with someone in the family, discuss it.

9. Get rest, or what I refer to as your "nappy poo."

10. Keep yourself looking nice. I lay my clothes out the night before. I always have my makeup on, a flower on my lapel, and nice ribbon to finish it off.

11. Bonus: A few days after visiting with Lucille, she called to say she left off the list what may be the most important thing: *Forgiveness.*

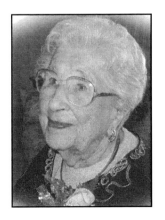

Anne Beversluis, 103 years old, Oceanside, California
Anne is a spunky 103-year-old-lady who is fun and laughs easily. Despite age's challenges, she is stylish, always bejeweled, in full makeup, and with hair perfectly coifed. She adores her family and lives a life of faith and integrity. She inspires everyone she meets with her grace and charm. Her favorite hymn is "Great Is Thy Faithfulness," as God is her source and comfort. In Anne's words:
"I have no magical secret as to how I achieved this blessed age, but I can tell you how I've lived my life:

1. I have a strong faith in God and His will and purpose for my life.

2. I read the Bible every day.

3. I pray constantly throughout the day.

4. I eat in moderation (have never been on a diet).

5. I go to bed early.

6. I find great joy and comfort in my family.

7. I try to live a life of kindness focused on others.

8. I get dressed everyday with my hair fixed, makeup and jewelry on.

9. I stay engaged by doing crossword puzzles, listening to the news, etc.

10. I don't let grief consume me, but give it its rightful place and then move on.

"I live with my oldest daughter and son-in-law. It's a blessing to be with family. Every day I get up around nine, get dressed, and put on my jewelry. My daughter fixes my hair and makeup. This helps me be cheerful and feeling good about myself, while setting a good example for my family. I have breakfast and make my bed, straighten up my room, and listen to books on DVD, or as I call them, my 'talking books.' I have difficulty with my vision, but this helps me keep up with my reading. After dinner I love to watch the shopping channel I and go to bed around nine."

"I am able to enjoy the wonderful California weather as I shop and run errands with my daughter. I also get to visit with my other daughter, her husband, son and his wife, and my latest little great-granddaughter who is four months old. My family is my joy."

"On Sundays I go to church and have become a surrogate mom to many of the members who no longer have their moms around. I am happy to be needed by so many at this age, which gives me purpose."

"I was blessed to be able to take care of my husband in our home after he became ill and nursed him until he passed away. I wanted him to know how much I loved him and wanted my children to see that marriage is a commitment for better or worse, and forever. Cherish each moment of life—it passes before you know it. I can't believe that I am 103 years old. My spirit soars with youth and vitality and zest for life, even though my body can't always keep up. Live in the moment and let God worry about the future. My final moments each day are spent talking to God, and I put my head on the pillow with contentment and peace knowing He has it all under control."

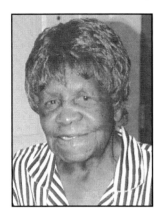

Julia Bethea (aka Mother Dear), 105 years, Toney, Alabama
Hailing from Toney, Alabama, Julia Bethea is 105 and going strong. Known affectionately by loved ones as "Mother Dear," this powerhouse can be seen on YouTube pumping iron at her local gym. She also enjoys cooking and working in her garden. Julia surrounds herself with friends and family who cherish her vibrant personality, wit, and loving disposition.

Mother Dear's top ten tips to live to 100:

1. Good nutrition: I eat a vegan diet full of fruits, vegetables, and grains. I try to limit grease and sweets.

2. Exercise: I work out at the gym and walk up and down the road in front of my home. You should keep moving, but know your limitations.

3. Prayer life: I petition the Lord in prayer and give thanksgiving and praise.

4. Sense of humor: I laugh at myself all of the time, especially around family and friends. I also like to make witty remarks.

5. Social life: I really enjoy being around people.

6. Read the Bible: I make it a daily habit to read my Bible.

7. Drink plenty of water: For the most part, I only drink water.

8. No alcohol, tobacco or soft drinks

9. Rest and good sleep habits: When I'm tired, I go to sleep. I don't try to force myself to stay awake to "hang out."

10. Outdoor activity for the air and sunlight: I love working in my garden and upkeeping my home.

Julia describes her daily routine:

"I like to keep active by working around the house, exercising, and staying involved in the senior ministries at my church. A couple of years ago, my daughter and adult grandchildren took me to buy a brand new computer. (They kept giving me their old ones and they kept breaking.) Now I use my new computer to search for healthy recipes online."

Note: Julia credits her longevity to her lifestyle as a Seventh-day Adventist. This religion is commonly associated with long and healthy lives. Refer back to Chapter 2 to learn more about which subcultures are living the longest.

THE YEAR 1907

Average life expectancy: 46 years

Average wage for a worker was 22 cents per hour. Annual income was $200–$400

The U.S. flag received its 46th star (Oklahoma)

Only 14% of homes in the United States had bathtubs

The United States only had 144 miles of paved roads

The maximum speed limit was 10 mph

Ninety percent of doctors did not have a college education—little wonder the average life expectancy was 46!

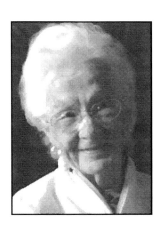

Helen Caylor, 100 years, Punxsutawney, Pennsylvania
Helen Caylor is a kind centenarian from Pennsylvania. Somewhat of a local celebrity, her independent spirit has attracted the attention of newspapers and email newsletters. She loves to quilt and has a voracious appetite for books, reading several a week. She believes in generosity and in the importance of a positive outlook on life, and shared the following with us:

1.   Be kind and have a good personality: My attitude is to always have a pleasant attitude towards everyone, rather than being irritable or crabby.

2.   Respect others and their ideas: I always think of helping somebody and giving them credit, instead of running them down. I never condemn, but I try to show that *I'm* living right. Because of my example, they may want to change.

3.   Don't criticize others: Always have a pleasant way about you—never an attitude that you're smarter than or know more than other people do.

4.   Have a lot of hobbies: The more hobbies I have, the more that I have to talk about. The more I do and create, the more I can expect to share.

5.   Help others: If I make something and I'm going to donate it to somebody, I don't expect to be paid back for it—because God'll reward me in some other way, often more than whatever I gave.

6.   Take your time at whatever you are doing: My mother always told me, "Never be in a rush to do anything. Always take your time to think about it, and you're better off because you don't make a mistake that way."

7.   Do a lot of reading: I believe that the more you read to keep your mind active, the more you learn, 'cause you learn by reading how some *other* people live. Like all the stories about the Amish down there in central Pennsylvania.

8.   Never quarrel with anybody: My advice is to always get along, regardless of whether the other person is right or wrong. You can think about their idea and tell them how to improve it, but do it in a way that won't upset them.

9. Keep your days full: Every day I have something I need to do. Being busy keeps your mind sharp.

10. Always be conservative: I don't buy anything I don't need. And I keep a record of everything I buy. Every bit of it, every *penny* that comes in and every penny that I spend. Every penny that I give away, too. I have a record of every *bit* of it.

"I usually wake up around seven-thirty or eight each morning. I make my breakfast: juice, cereal (oatmeal or dry cereal), a piece of toast, and coffee. Then I read my Bible for ten minutes to have God with me all day long."

"I straighten up the house and then I start working on quilting projects. I sew till dinnertime (lunchtime). Every hour I get up and walk around, but if I get tired, I lie down and read awhile. And the first thing you know—I'll fall asleep. Then I go back to quilting, and I can quilt a lot better!"

"After quilting, maybe I'll bake something—cupcakes or muffins or biscuits—to snack on in the evening. After supper, I'll read or crochet. I don't read during the day, there's no time for that in the daytime. I get ready for bed, but I don't go to bed until after the news is on. I usually go to bed around midnight or a little after. But if [laughs] I'm readin' a good book, I'll read till 3:00 a.m. Then when I go to bed, I won't get up till 10 or 11 in the morning, but then the days are—too short. And I don't *like* that."

CONCLUSION

After compiling data from both the youngest generation and the oldest one, we realized that we are born with an innate sense of what is required for survival and true happiness. Somewhere along the way, most people forget what's important in life. Maybe it's the bombardment of advertising, unhealthy habits that have become socially acceptable, or the lack of personal responsibility. Regardless of what the cause is for this derailment, we hope the pages of this book will help you find your way back to a healthier and happier lifestyle—one that is based on a personal desire to do better each day.

If every day is met with the longing for an improved lifestyle and that longing is transformed into positive actions, a longer and healthier life is there for the taking. We wish you well. Go about your journey knowing that you have personal cheerleaders behind you every step of the way. When you blow out 100 candles some day, we hope that part of your journey was paved by the inspiration we have provided.

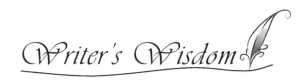

A BETTER MAN

Three months before my son Mathew was born, my father died from leukemia. He had worked his whole life as a laborer in an iron foundry, shoveling sand and pouring molten iron in the heat and smell of hell. He drank a bottle of whiskey and inhaled at least three packs of cigarettes a day. After a year of unsuccessful treatment, he was finally released from his suffering. He was no longer the strong man he used to be. In his last words, Tato (Ukrainian for Dad) begged me to read the Bible and to become a better man and father than he had been.

We buried my father on a cold winter day. His casket was lowered into that hardest of ground: the Canadian Tundra. Tears froze as fast as they were made.

The next season, Mathew, my son, was born on a glorious day in Texas. After months of grief, I finally had a reason to smile. I phoned family and friends with the good news. In just 24 hours, they greeted his arrival home with banners and gifts. His blue eyes captivated all, and after the celebrations ceased and the visitors left, he slept peacefully.

The next morning, I left to buy a video camera, wanting to capture all the memories that lie ahead. I returned to find him asleep in his warm bassinet. My late wife decided to awaken Mathew from his slumber and give him a sponge bath. She returned ashen-faced and said he was not breathing.

Rushing to him I could see that he was no longer a pink little baby, but was blue and lifeless. I placed him on our bed and commenced CPR. I called 911 between rescue breaths. It was surreal to be doing CPR on my own son.

The paramedics arrived and took over the mouth-to-mouth and chest compressions. They placed a breathing tube into Mathew and we were off in the ambulance. A throng of neighbors gawked as we made our way down the street. Inside the ambulance, I was in a daze as the paramedics fought to save my son's life. I remembered from my Catholic upbringing that in an emergency a doctor could baptize a dying person, so I baptized my son.

We pulled up to the emergency room of the hospital that Mathew had been born in just a day earlier. The doctors and nurses that took over his care were my friends. As everyone scattered to do their job, I was left alone in the middle of the ER in my tank top and tennis shoes, feeling for the first time as if I didn't belong there. Had I not been a doctor, I would have had all sorts of people from the hospital to console me, but they were all working; so instead, I was alone and I was scared.

Out of nowhere a doctor I vaguely knew was beside me. He was a recovered alcoholic whom I never referred patients to because of his drinking history. He comforted me, brought me coffee, and treated me like a son. He reminded me of my own father. After Mathew's mother arrived, he quickly disappeared. I never saw him again.

Mathew was lowered into the warm soft Texas soil on a sunny spring day. My tears watered the ground and sunk into the earth as fast as they hit it.

I was never the same after losing my father and my son. As a physician I had grown accustomed to seeing death, but now I had personally felt the indescribable pain I had seen on the countless faces of others over the years. For years after, I would cry for no reason, but out of the ashes of these tragedies was born a better doctor. Now it is my calling to help others live a long and healthy life, not just for themselves, but for those they may leave behind.

—Walter Gaman, MD

GENE MOORE, 90 YEARS YOUNG, ST. GEORGE, UTAH

He recently celebrated his 66th wedding anniversary. "A few things that help keep me active and healthy include jumping on the trampoline, 8 hours of sleep with a 20 minute nap, and keeping a positive attitude!"

ABOUT THE AUTHORS

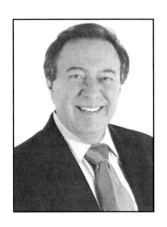

Walter Gaman, MD, is Board Certified and a Fellow of the American Board of Family Practice. As a seasoned professional and medical expert, he is a regular on Fox News Radio, as well as Good Morning Texas and other media outlets. In addition, Dr. Gaman co-hosts the nationally syndicated *Staying Young Radio Show*.

As a founding partner at Executive Medicine of Texas, Dr. Gaman's passion is to educate people on how they can be proactive about their health. He believes everyone has the ability to reach their 100th birthday, while still having a smile on their face and a skip in their step. It was this very passion for health that lead to Newsweek Magazine naming him as a "Best Doctor in Texas" in 2010, as well as numerous other accolades.

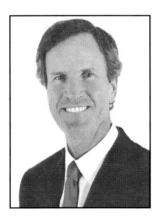

J. Mark Anderson, MD is Board Certified in Family Practice. Named a *HealthCare Hero 2013* by the Fort Worth Business Press, he has devoted his career to helping others reach their full health potential. His dedication to keeping up with the latest science and technology is what makes him one of the most sought after physicians in the country.

Dr. Anderson can be heard around the nation each week on The *Staying Young Radio Show*. As a much sought after health expert in the media, he has made a name for himself on both the local and national level with appearances on multitude of shows. Dr. Anderson is a regular guest on Fox News Radio as a top medical expert.

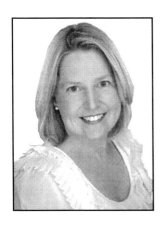

Judy Gaman, BSHS, CCRC is a health and wellness expert at Executive Medicine of Texas, as well as co-host on the nationally syndicated *Staying Young Radio Show.*

She graduated from The George Washington School of Medicine and Health Sciences with a degree in Clinical Research and has over 25 years of experience in the healthcare industry.

She is an award-winning published author with many titles to her name. She enjoys speaking to large groups and continues to empower individuals with health information and useful tips. Judy appears regularly in the media as a health and wellness expert, and is heard regularly across the nation as a Fox News Radio expert.

OTHER BOOKS:

Executive Medicine: Optimizing Your Chances for a Longer Life
Stay Young: 10 Proven Steps to Ultimate Health

BIBLIOGRAPHY

ABEL, E., KRUGER, M. (2009). "Smile Intensity in Photographs Predicts Longevity." *Psychological Science,* 21(4) 542–544. Retrieved from http://pss.sagepub.com/content/21/4/542

AFP. (2008). "HAPPINESS IS Key to Longevity." *The Sydney Morning Herald.* Retrieved from http://www.smh.com.au/lifestyle/diet-and-fitness/happiness-is-key-to-longevity-20090407-9y1p.html

AGARWAL, K. (MARCH 29, 2010). "Positive Attitude Helps You Keep Healthy—Study." TheMedGuru. Retrieved from http://www.themedguru.com/node/33551

ALLIANCE FOR AGING RESEARCH. (1999). "Can We Live Longer by Eating Fewer Calories?" Retrieved from http://agingresearch.org/content/article/detail/629

ARNOLD, L. (JUNE 30, 2012). "Live Life Fully: Could You Be Addicted to Stress?" *The Charleston Gazette.* Retrieved from http://wvgazette.com/Life/201206290113

BBC NEWS (OCTOBER 4 2006). "Cigars and Sex 'Boost Cuba Lives.'" Retrieved from http://news.bbc.co.uk/2/hi/americas/5407636.stm

BOYES, A., & DUGGAN, D. (July 27, 2009). "The Science of Being Happy." Mindfood.com. Retrieved from http://aliceboyes.com/MF0709-Happiness.pdf

BRIGHT REICH, J. (2008). "Healthy Choice: The 101 Best Things to Do For Your Body Now!" *Women's Health.* Retrieved from http://www.womenshealthmag.com/health/the-most-healthy-things-you-can-do

BYU IDAHO. (2006). "THE Tremendous Effects of a Positive Attitude." *On Wellness, 2*(4), 2. Retrieved from http://www2.byui.edu/CampusWellness/aprilprint.pdf

CAROLLO, K. (JUNE 5, 2012). "Centenarians' Positive Attitude Linked to Long Life." ABC News. Retrieved from http://abcnews.go.com/Health/centenarians-positive-attitude-linked-long-healthy-life/story?id=16494151

CENTERS FOR DISEASE CONTROL and Prevention. (2011). "Tobacco Use: Targeting the Nation's Leading Killer." Retrieved from http://www.cdc.gov/chronicdisease/resources/publications/aag/osh.htm

CENTERS FOR DISEASE CONTROL and Prevention. (2012). "Chronic Diseases and Health

Promotion." Retrieved from http://www.cdc.gov/chronicdisease/overview/index.htm

CENTERS FOR MEDICARE AND Medicaid Services, Office of the Actuary, National Health Statistics Group. (January 2012). "National Health Care Expenditures." http://www.cms.gov/Research-Statistics-Data-and-Systems/Statistics-Trends-and-Reports/NationalHealthExpendData/downloads/tables.pdf

CHAN, A. L. (2012). "Longer Learning Could Up Your Life Expectancy, Study Suggests." HuffPost Healthy Living. Retrieved from http://www.huffingtonpost.com/2012/05/16/longer-learning-life-expectancy-longevity_n_1521562.html

CHARLAP, S. (JUNE 5, 2012). "Why We Live Longer Is More Important Than How Long We Live." Retrieved from http://mdprevent.blogspot.com/2012/06/advantages-of-living-longer-right-way.html

CRAWFORD, B., LEVITT, E. B., & Newman, G. F. (2000). "Laughter Good for Heart." University of Maryland Medical Center. Retrieved from http://www.umm.edu/news/releases/laughter.htm

DEEPENDER, D. (OCTOBER 16, 2012). "Oldest Dad Becomes Father Again at 96." *Times of India*. Retrieved from http://articles.timesofindia.indiatimes.com/2012-10-16/india/34497611_1_oldest-man-nanu-ram-jogi-first-child

DUKE UNIVERSITY (MARCH 24, 2010). "People Are Living Longer and Healthier: Now What?" *Science Daily*. Retrieved from http://today.duke.edu/2010/03/aging.html

FENSTER, M. S. (SEPTEMBER 21, 2011). "We're Living Longer Than Ever Before, But Are We Healthier?" *The Atlantic*. Retrieved from http://www.theatlantic.com/health/archive/2011/09/were-living-longer-than-ever-before-but-are-we-healthier/245409/#

FOSSEL, M., BLACKBURN, G., & Woynarowski, D. (2011). *The Immortality Edge*. Hoboken, New Jersey: John Wiley & Sons, Inc.

FREEDMAN, N. D. (2012). "Association of Coffee Drinking with Total and Cause-Specific Mortality." *New England Journal of Medicine, 366,* 1891–1904. Retrieved from http://www.nejm.org/doi/full/10.1056/NEJMoa1112010

GASKELL, K. J. (MAY 17, 2010). "Tricks to Positive Thinking" Livestrong.com. Retrieved from http://www.livestrong.com/article/129583-tricks-positive-thinking/

GIULIANO, V. E. (2008). "Protection Against Radiation—The Second Line of Defense."

Bibliography

Retrieved from http://www.vincegiuliano.name/PROTECTION%20AGAINST%20RADIA-TIONc.htm

GUILLAMS, T. (1999). "HEALTHY Microbial Organisms." *The Standard*, 2, 1–7.

GUILLAMS, T. (MAY/JUNE 2000). "Fatty Acids: Essential…Therapeutic." *The Standard*, 3, 1–7.

GUILLAMS, T. (2001). "FEMALE Cycle Difficulties: Non-invasive Diagnosis and Natural Treatment Options." *The Standard*, 4, 1–7.

GUILLAMS, T. (2002). "DIABETES—THE Preventable Epidemic." *The Standard*, 5, 1–7.

GUILLAMS, T. (2004). "HOMOCYSTEINE—A Risk Factor for Vascular Diseases: Guidelines for Clinical Practice." *The Journal of the American Nutraceutical Association*, 7, 1–24.

HARVARD HEALTH. (JANUARY 25, 2012). "Positive Thinking Seems to Help the Heart." *Chicago Tribune*. Retrieved from http://articles.chicagotribune.com/2012-01-25/health/sc-health-0125-heart-study-20120125_1_heart-disease-positive-emotions-emotional-health

HEALTHISHBLOG.COM (JULY 28, 2011). "How a Positive Attitude Can Improve your Immune System." Retrieved from http://healthishblog.com/how-a-positive-attitude-can-improve-your-immune-system/

HERRINGTON, D. (JUNE 27, 2012). "13 Health Benefits of Pumpkin Seeds." Care 2. Retrieved from http://www.care2.com/greenliving/13-health-benefits-of-pumpkin-seeds.html

HOTZ, R. L. (JULY 1, 2010). "Scientists Discover Keys to Long Life." WSJ.com. Retrieved from http://online.wsj.com/article/SB10001424052748703571704575341034212066208.html

IPAKTCHIAN, S. (JUNE 7, 2010). "Medical School to Offer Course that Gives Students Option of Studying their Own Genotype Data." *Stanford Medicine*. Retrieved from http://med.stanford.edu/ism/2010/june/genotype.html

JASLOW, R. (JUNE 29, 2011). "New Study Is Wake-Up Call for Diet Soda Drinkers." *CBS News*. Retrieved from http://www.cbsnews.com/8301-504763_162-20075358-10391704/new-study-is-wake-up-call-for-diet-soda-drinkers/

JENNY, N. S. (JULY 2012). "Inflammation in Aging: Cause, Effect, or Both?" *Discovery Medicine*. Retrieved from http://www.discoverymedicine.com/Nancy-S-Jenny/2012/06/25/inflammation-in-aging-cause-effect-or-both/

JOHNS HOPKINS HEALTH ALERT. (August 3, 2011). "BPH Concerns: Does BPH Lead to Prostate Cancer?" Retrieved from http://www.johnshopkinshealthalerts.com/alerts/enlarged_prostate/BPH_5815-1.html

Klein, L. (2010). "11 Foods that Get your Sex Drive Going Naturally." *Organic Authority.* Retrieved from http://www.organicauthority.com/mojo-foods/11-foods-that-get-your-sex-drive-going-naturally.html

Koerth-Baker, M. (August 29, 2008). "The Power of Positive Thinking: Truth or Myth?" Live Science. Retrieved from http://www.livescience.com/2814-power-positive-thinking-truth-myth.html

Krach, C. A., & Velcoff, V. A. (July 1999). "Centenarians in the United States." U.S. Department of Health and Human Services. Retrieved from http://www.census.gov/prod/99pubs/p23-199.pdf

Low Glycemic Foods: Why Low Glycemic Diets are Better. (2010) *Natural Health Guide.* Retrieved from http://www.natural-health-guide.com

Mail Online. (July 6, 2011). "Dawn of a New Age: The First Person to Reach 150 Is Already Alive…And Soon We'll Live to Be a Thousand, Claims Scientist." Retrieved from http://www.dailymail.co.uk/sciencetech/article-2011425/The-person-reach-150-alive--soon-live-THOUSAND-claims-scientist.html

Martin, F. (August 31, 2010). "The Link Between Positive Psychology and Cancer Survival." *Highlight Health.* Retrieved from http://www.highlighthealth.com/research/the-link-between-positive-psychology-and-cancer-survival/

Martin-Kilgour, Z. (n.d.). "Benefits of a Positive Attitude [Even Outweigh a Healthy Diet for Longevity]." Secrets of Longevity in Humans. Retrieved from http://www.secrets-of-longevity-in-humans.com/benefits-of-a-positive-attitude.html

MedicineNet.com. (2006). "Life Extension: Science Fact or Science Fiction?" Retrieved from http://medicinenet.com/script/main/art.asp?articlekey=60659

MicroscopeMaster.com. (n.d.). "Nanobots: Uses in Medicine and Industry." Retrieved from http://www.microscopemaster.com/nanobots.html

Parenting.com. (2013). "12 Immunity-Boosting Snacks." *Parenting.* Retrieved from http://www.parenting.com/gallery/12-immunity-boosting-snacks?pnid=111524

Pelletier, D. "Medical Nanobots Could End Disease, Aging in 2 Decades." PositiveFuturist.com. Retrieved from http://www.positivefuturist.com/archive/334.html

PopSugar Fitness. (2009). "Glycemic Index: Where do Sweeteners Fall?" Retrieved from http://www.fitsugar.com/Glycemic-Index-Where-Do-Sweeteners-Fall-3031565

RIMER, S. (2011). "HAPPINESS and Health." *HSPH News.* Retrieved from www.hsph.harvard.edu/news/magazine/happiness-stress-heart-disease/

ROSENKILDE, M., ET AL. (2012). "Body Fat Loss and Compensatory Mechanisms in Response to Different Doses of Aerobic Exercise." *American Psychological Society.* Retrieved from http://ajpregu.physiology.org/content/early/2012/07/30/ajpregu.00141.2012.abstract

SAENZ, A. (AUGUST 26, 2009). "CDC Report: Americans Living Longer, But Not As Long As Everyone Else." *SingularityHub.* Retrieved from http://singularityhub.com/2009/08/26/cdc-report-americans-living-longer-but-not-as-long-as-everyone-else/

SCIENCEDAILY.COM. (MARCH 5, 2009). "Human Emotions Hold Sway over Physical Health Worldwide." *Science Daily.* Retrieved July 2, 2012, from http://www.sciencedaily.com/releases/2009/03/090304091229.htm

SCIENCEDAILY.COM. (SEPTEMBER 20, 2011). "Feed your Genes: How our Genes Respond to the Foods we Eat. ScienceDaily Science News. Retrieved from http://www.sciencedaily.com/releases/2011/09/110919073845.htm

SCOMMEGNA, P. (JULY 2011). "More of Us on Track to Reach Age 100: Genes, Habits, Baboons Examined for Longevity Clues." Population Reference Bureau. Retrieved from http://www.prb.org/Articles/2011/biodemography.aspx

SEGAL, R., SEGAL, J., & Smith, M. (2012). "Improving Emotional Health: Strategies and Tips for Good Mental Health." HelpGuide.org. Retrieved from http://www.helpguide.org/mental/mental_emotional_health.htm

SHAW, G. (FEBRUARY 2012). "The Right Type: Personal Genetic Testing in the Medical School Curriculum." Association of American Medical Colleges. Retrieved from https://www.aamc.org/newsroom/reporter/feb2012/273822/genetic-testing.html

SIMON, N. (MAY 13, 2011). "6 Ways to Feel Happier, Be Healthier." AARP Bulletin. Retrieved from http://www.aarp.org/health/healthy-living/info-05-2011/6-ways-to-feel-happier-be-healthier.html

SPECTRACELL LABORATORIES. (2012). "NUTRIENT Correlation Wheels: Deficiencies Correlated with Disease Conditions." [Brochure].

THE EMERGING RISK FACTORS Collaboration. (2011). "Diabetes Mellitus, Fasting Glucose, and Risk of Cause-Specific Death." *The New England Journal of Medicine*, 364, 829–841. Retrieved from http://www.nejm.org/doi/full/10.1056/NEJMoa1008862

Toole, M. "Laughter and Health: Laughter Is the Cure for All that Ails You." Healthy Holistic Living. Retrieved from http://www.healthy-holistic-living.com/Laughter-and-Health.html#ixzz28Xrqofyt

Wadley, J. (July 21, 2011). "Positive Thinking: Optimism Lowers Risk of Having Stroke." University of Michigan News Service. Retrieved from http://ns.umich.edu/new/releases/8486

Windsor, A. (n.d.). "Medicine Will Not Only Make Us Live Longer, But Live Better." Guardian.co.uk. Retrieved from http://www.guardian.co.uk/zurichfuturology/story/0,,1952688,00.html

Winterman, D. (February 19, 2008). "The Towns Where People Live the Longest." *BBC News*. Retrieved from http://news.bbc.co.uk/2/hi/uk_news/magazine/7250675.stm

Zelman, K. (2012). "15 Immune-Boosting Foods." WebMD. Retrieved from http://www.webmd.com/cold-and-flu/ss/slideshow-immune-foods